CPAP and Oxygen for Dementia

CPAP and Oxygen for Dementia

A Dementia Care Essentials Guide

PETER M. ABRAHAM, BSN, RN

This book and the Dementia Care Essentials series it is part of are dedicated to multiple parties that helped shape my experiences and wisdom in caring for loved ones suffering from various types of dementia. I've worked with loved ones with dementia in long-term care as a registered nurse supervisor and as a hospice case manager. Caregivers and family members provided the most significant insights over the years.

Deborah, the wife of an Alzheimer's hospice at-home patient, provided insight into how the brains of dementia patients can be thought of like an electric clock. Most of the time, the clock is short-circuited and, therefore, not working correctly, but at times, as the clock's hands turn, the short-circuit goes away. For a fleeting time, a day or so, the person appears as if they don't have dementia.

Kathy is one of four daughters of a dementia patient for whom I provided care in a memory care center raised thought-provoking questions about the ethical dilemma of waking loved ones with dementia who want to sleep all the time to feed them vs. just letting them sleep.

Linda, who worked alongside me with a dementia patient, a former registered nurse herself, helped me understand other applications of validation therapy (a set of strategies and techniques that will be discussed in this book), such as rolling with resistance, which included accepting the nickname of "Jack," rather than my desire to be called Peter.

Jed, for whom I cared for his mother at home and then within a memory care center, reminded me of the actual cost that cannot be measured in terms of money of being a family caregiver.

Then there's our family journey, where my mother-in-law developed mixed dementia -- Alzheimer's disease plus vascular dementia – and was being cared for at home by her late husband, and then in a memory care center after he died suddenly.

More family members are involved, each helping me gain wisdom not taught in books. It is to all of these families and caregivers, as well as my late mother-in-law, Loris, and my wife, Laura, to whom this book and the others in this series are dedicated.

Table of Contents

Introduction

I know caring for someone with dementia can be challenging, especially when your loved one should be wearing external oxygen or using a CPAP at night. As an experienced nurse who's worked in long-term care and hospice, I've seen firsthand how difficult it can be for families and caregivers.

Taking care of a loved one with dementia is already a big task. They might not even realize they have dementia, which can make things even trickier. It's like they're moving forward in time physically, but mentally and emotionally, and functionally, they're heading back to being entirely dependent, kind of like a newborn.

That's why I wanted to write this book. I hope it'll give you some helpful strategies for encouraging your loved one with dementia to wear oxygen if needed, use their CPAP at night, or both. And don't worry—many of these tips will also benefit other aspects of caregiving!

I've set up this book with you in mind. We'll start by discussing why it's so crucial for you to take care of yourself. When someone you love has a serious, long-term illness like dementia (which can last for decades), it affects the whole family. The person with dementia isn't the only one suffering - caregivers like you are going through a lot, too.

After we cover self-care and some practical tips, we will discuss the importance of early legal and financial planning, which is crucial to protect yourself and your loved one. Then, we'll discuss validation therapy and other ways to communicate better with your loved one. Trust me, these skills will come in handy in all sorts of tricky situations, not just with dementia care.

Once we've got those basics down, we'll get into the nitty-gritty of encouraging the use of external oxygen and wearing the CPAP at night for someone with dementia. And since many people with dementia eventually need end-of-life care, we'll wrap up by covering that vital topic, too.

I'm here to help you through this journey. It isn't easy, but you can do it with the right tools and support. Remember, you're not alone in this!

Caring for the Caregiver

Caring for a loved one with dementia is a journey of profound love and dedication, but it's also one of the most challenging roles a person can undertake. As caregivers and family members, you stand at the forefront of this complex and often overwhelming experience. Your commitment to providing compassionate care is admirable, yet it's crucial to recognize the significant impact this role can have on your well-being.

The Emotional and Physical Toll

The path of a dementia caregiver is paved with a myriad of emotions and physical demands that can test even the strongest individuals. Let's explore the multifaceted nature of this toll:

Emotional Challenges:

1. Grief and loss: Watching a loved one's cognitive decline

2. Guilt: Feeling inadequate or struggling with difficult decisions

3. Anxiety: Worrying about the future and managing daily uncertainties

4. Frustration: Dealing with repetitive behaviors and communication barriers

5. Isolation: Experiencing a shrinking social circle and loss of personal time

Physical Demands:

- Sleep deprivation due to irregular sleep patterns of the care recipient

- Chronic stress leading to weakened immune function

- Neglect of personal health needs and medical appointments

- Physical strain from assisting with mobility and personal care tasks

- Exhaustion from constant vigilance and round-the-clock care

These emotional and physical challenges create a complex web that can entangle even the most resilient caregivers. It's essential to recognize that experiencing these difficulties doesn't reflect on your capabilities or dedication – it's a natural response to an extraordinarily demanding situation.

Common Caregiver Emotions	Physical Manifestations	Potential Long-term Consequences
Sadness, Grief	Fatigue, Weakened Immunity	Depression, Chronic Illness
Anxiety, Worry	Insomnia, Muscle Tension	Anxiety Disorders, Chronic Pain
Frustration, Anger	High Blood Pressure, Headaches	Cardiovascular Issues, Migraines
Guilt, Self-doubt	Appetite Changes, Digestive Issues	Eating Disorders, Gastrointestinal Problems

Recognizing the Signs of Caregiver Burnout

Caregiver burnout is a state of physical, emotional, and mental exhaustion that can creep up slowly or suddenly. Awareness of the warning signs is crucial to prevent reaching this critical point. Here are key indicators to watch for:

1. **Emotional Signs:**

   o   Feeling overwhelmed or constantly worried

   o   Experiencing mood swings or irritability

   o   Losing interest in activities once enjoyed

   o   Feeling hopeless, helpless, or alone

2. **Physical Signs:**

- o   Frequently falling ill or feeling constantly tired
- o   Changes in appetite or sleep patterns
- o   Neglecting personal hygiene or appearance
- o   Developing new health problems or exacerbating existing ones

3. **Behavioral Signs:**

- o   Withdrawing from friends and family
- o   Procrastinating on important tasks
- o   Using alcohol, food, or medications to cope
- o   Lashing out at the person with dementia or others

4. **Cognitive Signs:**

- o   Difficulty concentrating or making decisions
- o   Forgetfulness in daily tasks
- o   Trouble problem-solving or thinking clearly
- o   Negative thought patterns or constant worry

Self-Assessment Checklist for Caregiver Burnout:

Warning Sign	Frequency (Rarely/Sometimes/Often/Always)
I feel exhausted even after sleeping.	
I catch myself yelling or arguing more often.	
I've stopped seeing friends or engaging in hobbies.	
I feel resentful towards the person I'm caring for.	
I worry constantly about the future.	
I neglect my own health needs.	
I have trouble falling asleep or staying asleep.	
I feel like I can't do anything right.	

If you find yourself answering "Often" or "Always" to several of these statements, it may be time to seek additional support and focus on self-care strategies.

Remember, recognizing these signs is not an admission of failure but a crucial step in maintaining your ability to provide care. By acknowledging the challenges and being vigilant about your well-being, you can take proactive steps to prevent burnout and ensure that you can continue to provide the best possible care for your loved one with dementia. Your role is invaluable, and by taking care of yourself, you're also ensuring the best care for your loved one.

Understanding the Importance of Self-Care

As caregivers and family members supporting individuals with dementia, you're intimately familiar with the concept of care. However, it's crucial to remember that care must also extend to you. Self-care isn't a luxury; it's a necessity that directly impacts your ability to provide compassionate, practical support to your loved ones or patients.

The Impact of Self-Care on Caregiving Quality

The quality of care you provide is intrinsically linked to your well-being. When you prioritize self-care, you benefit yourself and enhance your capacity to care for others. Let's explore how self-care positively influences various aspects of caregiving:

1. **Enhanced Emotional Resilience**

    o Better equipped to handle stress and emotional challenges

    o Increased patience and empathy in difficult situations

    o Improved ability to maintain a calm demeanor

2. **Improved Physical Stamina**

    o Greater energy to perform caregiving tasks

    o Reduced risk of caregiver-related injuries

    o Increased overall health, leading to fewer sick days

3. **Sharpened Mental Acuity**

    o Better decision-making skills in critical situations

    o Improved memory and attention to detail

    o Enhanced problem-solving abilities

4. **Strengthened Relationships**

    o more positive interactions with the care recipient

- o Healthier boundaries with family members and healthcare professionals

- o Improved communication skills

5. **Increased Caregiving Longevity**

- o Reduced risk of burnout and compassion fatigue

- o Sustained ability to provide care over extended periods

- o Greater job satisfaction for professional caregivers

Self-Care Practice	Benefits to Caregiver	Impact on Caregiving Quality
Regular Exercise	Improved physical health, stress relief	Increased energy, better mood during care
Adequate Sleep	Better cognitive function, emotional stability	Enhanced decision-making, patience in care
Mindfulness/Meditation	Reduced anxiety, improved focus	Increased presence and empathy in interactions
Social Connections	Emotional support, reduced isolation	Renewed energy and perspective in caregiving

Overcoming Guilt and Prioritizing Personal Needs

One of the most significant barriers to self-care for caregivers is the pervasive feeling of guilt. It's common to feel that taking time for yourself is selfish or detracts from the care you should provide. However, overcoming this guilt is essential for sustainable caregiving. Here's how to reframe your thinking and prioritize your needs:

Understanding Guilt in Caregiving:

- Recognize that guilt is a common and normal emotion for caregivers

- Acknowledge that guilt often stems from unrealistic expectations of yourself

- Realize that neglecting your needs can lead to resentment and diminished care quality

Strategies for Overcoming Caregiver Guilt:

1. **Reframe Your Perspective**

    o View self-care as a necessary part of providing good care

    o Understand that taking care of yourself allows you to be more present and effective

    o Recognize that you're modeling healthy behavior for others

2. **Set Realistic Expectations**

    o Accept that you can't do everything perfectly

    o Understand that it's okay to have limits and boundaries

    o Recognize that asking for help is a sign of strength, not weakness

3. **Practice Self-Compassion**

    o Treat yourself with the same kindness you show to others

    o Acknowledge your efforts and successes, no matter how small

    o Use positive self-talk to counter guilty thoughts

4. **Educate Yourself and Others**

   - o   Learn about the importance of self-care in caregiving literature

   - o   Share information with family members to gain their support

   - o   Discuss the benefits of caregiver well-being with healthcare professionals

5. **Start Small and Build**

   - o   Begin with short periods of self-care to ease into the practice

   - o   Gradually increase the time and frequency of self-care activities

   - o   Celebrate each step you take towards prioritizing your needs

Practical Steps to Prioritize Personal Needs:

- **Schedule Self-Care**: Block out time in your calendar for activities that rejuvenate you

- **Create a Self-Care Plan**: Develop a written plan outlining your self-care goals and strategies

- **Communicate Your Needs**: Clearly express your needs to family members and support networks

- **Use Respite Care**: Take advantage of respite services to get regular breaks

- **Join Support Groups**: Connect with other caregivers who understand your challenges

- **Seek Professional Help**: Consider therapy or counseling to work through feelings of guilt

Common Guilt-Inducing Thoughts	Reframed Perspective
"I should be doing more."	"I'm doing my best, and that's enough."
"Taking a break is selfish."	"Taking care of myself helps me provide better care."
"Nobody else can care for them like I can."	"Accepting help allows for fresh energy in caregiving."
"I don't deserve to enjoy myself."	"My well-being is important and valid."

Remember, prioritizing your needs isn't selfish—it's essential. You can continue providing the high-quality, compassionate care that your loved ones or patients deserve by taking care of yourself. Self-care is integral to the caregiving journey, benefiting you and those you care for. Embrace it without guilt, knowing that you're making a wise investment in your ability to care for others.

Physical Self-Care Strategies

Your physical health is the foundation of your ability to provide care as a caregiver. While putting your needs last is easy, maintaining your physical well-being is crucial for you and your loved one. Let's explore practical strategies to keep your body healthy and energized.

Maintaining a Healthy Diet

A nutritious diet is essential for sustaining your energy levels and overall health. Here are some strategies to ensure you're fueling your body properly:

1. **Plan and Prepare Meals in Advance**

    o   Use weekends or less busy times to batch-cook meals

    o   Freeze portions for easy reheating during hectic days

    o   Prepare healthy snacks to avoid reaching for processed foods

2. **Focus on Nutrient-Dense Foods**

- o Incorporate a variety of colorful fruits and vegetables

- o Choose whole grains over refined carbohydrates

- o Include lean proteins like fish, poultry, beans, and nuts

- o Don't forget healthy fats from sources like avocados and olive oil

3. **Stay Hydrated**

- o Keep a water bottle with you throughout the day

- o Set reminders to drink water regularly

- o Include hydrating foods like cucumbers and watermelon in your diet

4. **Mindful Eating**

- o Take time to sit down and enjoy your meals

- o Avoid eating while multitasking or when stressed

- o Listen to your body's hunger and fullness cues

5. **Seek Support**

- o Ask family members or friends to help with meal preparation

- o Consider meal delivery services for fresh, healthy options

- o Consult a nutritionist for personalized dietary advice if needed

Meal Type	Quick and Healthy Options
Breakfast	Greek yogurt with berries and nuts, overnight oats, whole grain toast with avocado.
Lunch	Mixed green salad with grilled chicken, whole grain wrap with hummus and vegetables.
Dinner	Baked salmon with roasted vegetables, vegetarian chili, stir-fry with tofu and mixed veggies.
Snacks	Apple slices with almond butter, carrot sticks with hummus, and a handful of mixed nuts.

Incorporating Regular Exercise

Exercise is not just about physical fitness; it's a powerful stress reliever and mood booster. Here's how to make physical activity a regular part of your routine:

1. **Find Activities You Enjoy**

   o Experiment with different types of exercise to find what you like

   o Consider activities that can involve your loved one, like gentle walks

   o Try yoga or tai chi for both physical and mental benefits

2. **Set Realistic Goals**

   o Start small. Even 10 minutes a day can make a difference

   o Gradually increase duration and intensity as you build stamina

   o Celebrate your progress, no matter how small

3. **Make It Convenient**

   o   Keep exercise equipment at home for quick workouts

   o   Use online fitness videos for guided sessions

   o   Take advantage of small pockets of time throughout the day

4. **Incorporate Movement into Daily Tasks**

   o   Do calf raises while washing dishes

   o   Perform stretches during TV commercials

   o   Take the stairs instead of the elevator when possible

5. **Seek Support and Accountability**

   o   Join a caregiver fitness group or online community

   o   Use fitness apps to track your progress

   o   Ask a friend or family member to be your exercise buddy

Exercise Type	Benefits	Caregiver-Friendly Examples
Cardiovascular	Improves heart health, boosts energy	Brisk walking, dancing, stationary cycling
Strength Training	Builds muscle, supports bone health	Bodyweight exercises, resistance bands, light dumbbells
Flexibility	Reduces muscle tension, improves mobility	Gentle stretching, yoga, tai chi
Balance	Prevents falls, improves stability	Single-leg stands, heel-to-toe walk, balance board

Ensuring Adequate Sleep and Rest

Quality sleep is crucial for your physical and mental well-being. Here are strategies to improve your sleep habits:

1. **Establish a Consistent Sleep Schedule**

   o   Try to go to bed and wake up at the same time each day

   o   Create a relaxing bedtime routine to signal your body it's time to sleep

   o   Avoid screens for at least an hour before bedtime

2. **Optimize Your Sleep Environment**

   o   Keep your bedroom cool, dark, and quiet

   o   Invest in a comfortable mattress and pillows

   o   Use white noise or earplugs if needed to block out disturbances

3. **Manage Nighttime Caregiving**

   o   Use night lights to avoid fully waking up for nighttime checks

   o   Consider assistive devices like bed alarms to alert you when needed

   o   Take turns with other family members for nighttime care if possible

4. **Practice Relaxation Techniques**

   o   Try deep breathing exercises before bed

   o   Use guided imagery or meditation to calm your mind

   o   Practice progressive muscle relaxation to release physical tension

5. **Be Mindful of Diet and Exercise**

  - Avoid caffeine and heavy meals close to bedtime

  - Exercise regularly, but not too close to bedtime

  - Limit alcohol, as it can disrupt sleep patterns

6. **Prioritize Rest During the Day**

  - Take short power naps (15-20 minutes) when possible

  - Use respite care to get a whole night's sleep occasionally

  - Practice mindfulness or meditation for mental rest during the day

Sleep Challenge	Potential Solution
Difficulty falling asleep	Practice a calming bedtime routine, and try relaxation techniques.
Waking up during the night	Keep a notepad by your bed to jot down thoughts, and use white noise.
Early morning wakings	Ensure your room is dark, and consider adjusting your sleep schedule.
Feeling unrested after sleep	Evaluate your sleep environment and consult a doctor about sleep quality.

Remember, taking care of your physical health is not selfish—it's a necessary part of being an effective caregiver. By prioritizing your diet, exercise, and sleep, you're ensuring you have the strength and energy to provide the best care possible for your loved one. Start with small, manageable changes, and be patient with yourself as you develop these healthy habits. Your body—and your loved one—will thank you for it.

Emotional and Mental Well-being

As a caregiver, tending to your emotional and mental health is just as crucial as maintaining your physical well-being. The demands of caring for a loved one can significantly toll your psychological state, making it essential to develop strategies that nurture your inner self. Let's explore some effective methods to support your emotional and mental well-being.

Practicing Mindfulness and Meditation

Mindfulness and meditation are powerful tools for managing stress, improving focus, and cultivating inner peace. These practices can be particularly beneficial for caregivers, offering moments of calm in challenging situations.

Benefits of Mindfulness and Meditation for Caregivers:

- Reduced stress and anxiety

- Improved emotional regulation

- Enhanced ability to focus and concentrate

- Increased self-awareness and empathy

- Better sleep quality

- Boosted immune function

How to Incorporate Mindfulness and Meditation into Your Daily Routine:

1. **Start Small**

    - Begin with just 5 minutes a day

    - Gradually increase the duration as you become more comfortable

2. **Choose a Consistent Time and Place**

    - Set aside a specific time each day for your practice

    - Create a quiet, comfortable space for meditation

3. **Explore Different Techniques**

   o   Try guided meditations using apps or online resources

   o   Experiment with breathing exercises, body scans, or loving-kindness meditation

   o   Practice mindful activities like walking or eating

4. **Be Patient and Non-Judgmental**

   o   Remember that it's normal for your mind to wander

   o   Gently bring your attention back to your focus point without self-criticism

5. **Integrate Mindfulness into Daily Activities**

   o   Practice being fully present during routine tasks like washing dishes or folding laundry

   o   Take mindful breaks throughout the day, even if just for a few deep breaths

Mindfulness Technique	Description	When to Use
Breath Awareness	Focus on the sensation of breathing, noticing each inhale and exhale	Any time, especially during stressful moments
Body Scan	Systematically relax each part of your body from head to toe	Before bed or during breaks
Loving-Kindness Meditation	Direct positive thoughts and wishes towards yourself and others	When feeling overwhelmed or frustrated
Mindful Walking	Pay attention to each step and your surroundings while walking	During outdoor breaks or while moving between tasks

Journaling and Emotional Expression

Journaling is a powerful tool for processing emotions, gaining clarity, and fostering self-reflection. For caregivers, it can serve as a private outlet for expressing the complex feelings often accompanying caregiving.

Benefits of Journaling for Caregivers:

- Emotional release and stress reduction
- Increased self-awareness and problem-solving
- Documentation of caregiving journey and memories
- Opportunity for a gratitude practice
- Improved communication skills

Tips for Effective Journaling:

1. **Choose Your Medium**

   - Traditional pen and paper
   - Digital journaling apps or word processors
   - Audio recordings or voice memos

2. **Set Aside Regular Time**

   - Aim for consistency, even if it's just a few minutes daily
   - Choose a time when you're least likely to be interrupted

3. **Write Freely Without Judgment**

   - Don't worry about grammar, spelling, or structure
   - Let your thoughts flow without censoring yourself

4. **Use Prompts When Needed**

- o "Today, I felt..."

- o "I'm grateful for..."

- o "A challenge I faced today was..."

- o "Something I learned about myself is..."

5. **Reflect on Your Entries**

- o Periodically review your journal to observe patterns and growth

- o Use insights gained to inform your self-care and caregiving strategies

6. **Explore Different Journaling Techniques**

- o Gratitude journaling

- o Stream of consciousness writing

- o Dialogue journaling (writing conversations with yourself or others)

- o Art journaling (combining writing with visual elements)

Journaling Method	Description	Benefit for Caregivers
Gratitude Journal	Daily list of things you're thankful for	Shifts focus to positive aspects of caregiving
Emotional Release Writing	Unfiltered expression of feelings and thoughts	Helps process difficult emotions and experiences
Problem-Solving Journal	Writing out challenges and brainstorming solutions	Enhances coping skills and decision-making
Reflection Journal	Regular entries about personal growth and insights	Promotes self-awareness and resilience

Seeking Professional Mental Health Support

While self-care practices are essential, there may be times when professional support is necessary. Seeking help from a mental health professional is a sign of strength and can provide valuable tools for managing the emotional challenges of caregiving.

Signs You May Benefit from Professional Support:

- Persistent feelings of sadness, anxiety, or hopelessness

- Difficulty managing anger or frustration

- Feeling overwhelmed or unable to cope

- Changes in sleep patterns or appetite

- Loss of interest in activities you once enjoyed

- Thoughts of self-harm or suicide

Types of Professional Mental Health Support:

1. **Individual Therapy**

   - One-on-one sessions with a licensed therapist or counselor.

   - Can focus on specific caregiving challenges or broader emotional issues.

2. **Support Groups**

   - Facilitated groups for caregivers to share experiences and coping strategies.

   - It can be in-person or online.

3. **Cognitive Behavioral Therapy (CBT)**

   - It helps identify and change negative thought patterns and behaviors.

   - It is particularly effective for managing anxiety and depression.

4. **Mindfulness-Based Stress Reduction (MBSR)**

   o Combines mindfulness meditation and yoga to reduce stress.

   o Often offered in 8-week programs.

5. **Telehealth Options**

   o Virtual therapy sessions via video call or phone.

   o Convenient for caregivers with limited time or transportation.

Steps to Access Mental Health Support:

1. **Consult Your Primary Care Physician**

   o Discuss your concerns and get referrals to mental health professionals.

2. **Check with Your Insurance Provider**

   o Understand your coverage for mental health services.

   o Get a list of in-network providers.

3. **Research Local Resources**

   o Contact local hospitals or community centers for caregiver support programs.

   o Look into non-profit organizations specializing in your loved one's condition.

4. **Consider Online Platforms**

   o Explore reputable online therapy services.

   o Look for platforms that offer specific support for caregivers.

5. **Don't Hesitate to Try Different Options**

- o   Switching therapists is okay if you don't feel a good connection.

- o   Explore different types of therapy to find what works best for you.

Type of Support	Best For	Potential Drawbacks
Individual Therapy	Personalized attention, deep exploration of issues	It can be costly, time-consuming
Support Groups	Shared experiences, practical advice from peers	Less individual focus and may not address specific needs
Online Therapy	Convenience, flexibility in scheduling	Potential technology issues, less personal connection
Crisis Hotlines	Immediate support during acute stress or emergencies	Not suitable for ongoing, in-depth support

Remember, taking care of your emotional and mental well-being is not a luxury—it's a necessity. By practicing mindfulness, journaling, and seeking professional support when needed, you're investing in your ability to provide compassionate care. Be patient with yourself as you explore these strategies, and remember that it's okay to prioritize your mental health. A mentally healthy caregiver is better equipped to face the challenges of caregiving with resilience and grace.

Building a Support Network

As a caregiver, it's crucial to remember that you don't have to face this journey alone. Building a solid support network can provide emotional support, practical assistance, and valuable resources. Let's explore how you can create and nurture a network that will sustain you through the challenges of caregiving.

Joining Caregiver Support Groups

Caregiver support groups offer a unique opportunity to connect with others who truly understand your experiences. These groups can be invaluable sources of emotional support, practical advice, and camaraderie.

Benefits of Joining Caregiver Support Groups:

- Emotional validation and understanding
- Sharing of practical tips and resources
- Reduced feelings of isolation and loneliness
- Opportunity to help others and feel empowered
- Access to educational resources and expert speakers

Types of Caregiver Support Groups:

1. **In-Person Groups**
   - Often held at community centers, hospitals, or religious organizations
   - Provide face-to-face interaction and immediate support

2. **Online Forums and Groups**
   - Accessible from anywhere, at any time
   - Offer anonymity and convenience

3. **Condition-Specific Groups**
   - Focus on caregivers dealing with particular illnesses or conditions
   - Provide specialized information and understanding

4. **Demographic-Specific Groups**
   - Cater to specific caregiver demographics (e.g., spouses, adult children, young caregivers)
   - Address unique challenges faced by different caregiver populations

How to Find and Join a Support Group:

1. Research local options through hospitals, community centers, or disease-specific organizations

2. Explore online platforms like Facebook groups or caregiver-specific websites

3. Ask your healthcare provider for recommendations

4. Consider starting your group if you can't find one that meets your needs

Type of Group	Pros	Cons
In-Person	Personal connection, immediate support	Time commitment, transportation needed
Online	Convenient, accessible 24/7	Lack of face-to-face interaction
Condition-Specific	Targeted advice, shared experiences	It may be limited in availability
General Caregiver	Broader perspective, diverse experiences	May lack specificity for your situation

Involving Family and Friends

Your existing network of family and friends can be a powerful source of support. However, many caregivers struggle with asking for help or feel guilty about burdening others. Remember, most people want to help but may not know how.

Strategies for Involving Family and Friends:

1. **Be Specific About Your Needs**

    o   Create a list of tasks that others can help with

    o   Be clear about what kind of support you're looking for (practical, emotional, etc.)

2. **Use Technology to Coordinate**

   o   Utilize care coordination apps or shared calendars

   o   Set up a group chat or email thread for updates and requests

3. **Educate Them About Your Caregiving Situation**

   o   Share information about your loved one's condition

   o   Help them understand the challenges you face

4. **Foster Ongoing Connections**

   o   Schedule regular check-ins or social gatherings

   o   Encourage friends and family to maintain a relationship with your care recipient

5. **Express Gratitude**

   o   Thank helpers for their support, no matter how small

   o   Let them know the positive impact of their assistance

Overcoming Barriers to Asking for Help:

- Recognize that accepting help benefits both you and your care recipient

- Start small if you're uncomfortable asking for big favors

- Remember that people often want to help but don't know how

Practice asking for help to become more comfortable with it Type of Support	Examples	How to Ask
Practical Assistance	Meal preparation, house cleaning, errands	"Could you pick up groceries for us this week?"
Respite Care	Sitting with the care recipient, overnight care	"Can you stay with Mom for a few hours on Saturday?"
Emotional Support	Listening, checking in, offering encouragement	"I'm having a tough week. Could we chat over coffee?"
Financial Help	Assistance with bills, fundraising	"We're struggling with medical expenses. Can you help us set up a fundraiser?"

Utilizing Community Resources and Respite Care

Community resources and respite care services can provide crucial support, allowing you to take breaks and access specialized assistance. These resources can help prevent burnout and ensure better care for you and your loved one.

Types of Community Resources:

1. **Area Agencies on Aging (AAA)**

    o Provide information, referrals, and sometimes direct services

    o Often offer caregiver support programs and resources

2. **Local Senior Centers**

  o May offer adult daycare programs

  o Provide social activities and meals for seniors

3. **Faith-Based Organizations**

  o Often have volunteer programs to assist caregivers

  o May offer support groups or counseling services

4. **Non-Profit Organizations**

  o Condition-specific organizations often have local chapters with resources

  o May offer educational workshops, support groups, or financial assistance

Respite Care Options:

1. **In-Home Respite**

  o Professional caregivers come to your home

  o Can range from a few hours to overnight care

2. **Adult Day Centers**

  o Provide care and activities during daytime hours

  o Often include meals and social interaction for care recipients

3. **Residential Respite**

  o Short-term stays at assisted living facilities or nursing homes

  o Allows for extended breaks or travel

4. **Volunteer Respite Programs**

  o Often run by community organizations or faith groups

  o May offer limited hours of free care

Steps to Access Community Resources and Respite Care:

1. Contact your local AAA for a comprehensive list of resources

2. Speak with your loved one's healthcare provider for recommendations

3. Research condition-specific organizations for specialized support

4. Explore online directories of senior services and respite care options

5. Consult with a social worker or case manager for personalized guidance

Resource Type	Services Offered	How to Access
Area Agency on Aging	Information, referrals, caregiver support programs	Call the local office or visit the website
Adult Day Centers	Daytime care, activities, meals	Contact the center directly for a tour and assessment
Home Health Agencies	In-home care, nursing services, respite	Get a referral from a doctor or contact an agency
Volunteer Programs	Companionship, errands, light housekeeping	Contact local senior centers or faith organizations

Remember, building a strong support network is an ongoing process. Finding the right combination of support groups, family involvement, and community resources that work for you may take time. Be patient with yourself and persistent in seeking out the help you need. By creating a robust support system, you're taking care of yourself and ensuring you can provide the best possible care for your loved one.

Don't hesitate to reach out and accept help when it's offered. Your role as a caregiver is invaluable, and by taking care of yourself through building a strong support network, you're ensuring that you can continue to provide compassionate care for the long term.

Time Management and Organization

As a caregiver, you often juggle multiple responsibilities, making time management and organization crucial skills. Effective planning can help reduce stress, increase efficiency, and ensure you and your loved one receive the care and attention needed. Let's explore strategies to help you manage your time and effectively organize your caregiving duties.

Creating a Caregiving Schedule

A well-structured caregiving schedule can provide a sense of routine and predictability, which benefits both you and your care recipient. Here's how to create an effective caregiving schedule:

1. **Assess Care Needs**

    - List all daily, weekly, and monthly tasks required for your loved one's care.

    - Include medical appointments, medication times, and personal care routines.

2. **Prioritize Tasks**

    - Identify critical tasks that must be done at specific times.

    - Determine which tasks are flexible and can be rescheduled if needed.

3. **Create a Template**

    - Use a digital calendar or a large paper calendar.

    - Color-code different types of activities for easy visualization.

4. **Include Self-Care**

    - Schedule time for your appointments, breaks, and activities.

    - Block out time for sleep and regular meals.

5. **Be Realistic**

- o Allow extra time for tasks, as caregiving often takes longer than expected.

- o Build buffer time for unexpected events or emergencies.

6. **Review and Adjust Regularly**

- o Reassess the schedule weekly or monthly.

- o Make changes as care needs evolve or your situation changes.

Time	Task	Responsible Person
7:00 AM	Morning medications and breakfast	Primary Caregiver
9:00 AM	Personal care and dressing	Home Health Aide
11:00 AM	Physical therapy exercises	Primary Caregiver
1:00 PM	Lunch and afternoon medications	Family Member
3:00 PM	Social activity or rest	Volunteer Companion
6:00 PM	Dinner and evening medications	Primary Caregiver
8:00 PM	Bedtime routine	Primary Caregiver

Delegating Tasks and Accepting Help

Delegating tasks and accepting help are essential for maintaining your well-being and ensuring comprehensive care for your loved one. Here's how to approach delegation effectively:

1. **Identify Delegable Tasks**

- o Make a list of tasks that don't require your specific expertise.

- o Consider which tasks others might enjoy or be well-suited to perform.

2. **Match Tasks to Helpers**

   o Consider the skills, availability, and preferences of potential helpers.

   o Assign tasks that align with each person's strengths and schedules.

3. **Communicate Clearly**

   o Provide detailed instructions for each task.

   o Set clear expectations for how and when tasks should be completed.

4. **Express Appreciation**

   o Thank helpers for their contributions, no matter how small.

   o Acknowledge the positive impact of their assistance.

5. **Be Open to Different Methods**

   o Recognize that others may complete tasks differently than you would.

   o Focus on results rather than specific methods when possible.

6. **Overcome Reluctance to Delegate**

   o Remind yourself that accepting help benefits both you and your loved one.

   o Start small if you're uncomfortable with extensive delegation.

Strategies for Effective Delegation:

- Use a shared task list or care coordination app.

- Rotate responsibilities among family members.

- Consider hiring professional help for specialized tasks.

- Utilize volunteer services for non-medical assistance.

Task Category	Examples	Potential Delegates
Household Chores	Cleaning, laundry, yard work	Family members, hired help, volunteers
Errands	Grocery shopping, pharmacy runs	Friends, neighbors, delivery services
Personal Care	Bathing, dressing, grooming	Home health aides, trained family members
Social Support	Companionship, activities	Friends, volunteers, adult day programs
Medical Management	Medication reminders, doctor appointments	Nursing services, tech solutions, family members

Using Technology to Streamline Caregiving Duties

Technology can be a powerful ally in managing caregiving responsibilities. Various tools can help simplify your caregiving journey, from organizing tasks to monitoring health. Here's how to leverage technology effectively:

1. **Care Coordination Apps**

   o Use apps designed for caregivers to manage schedules, tasks, and communication.

   o Examples: Caring Village, Lotsa Helping Hands, and CaringBridge.

2. **Medication Management Tools**

   o Utilize apps or smart pill dispensers to track and remind about medications.

   o Consider: Medisafe, PillPack, and Hero.

3. **Health Monitoring Devices**

   o   Implement wearable devices or smart home sensors for health tracking.

   o   Options: Fall detection devices, blood pressure monitors, GPS trackers.

4. **Communication Tools**

   o   Use video calling apps to connect with your loved one and other caregivers.

   o   Try: Skype, FaceTime, or Zoom.

5. **Online Support and Education**

   o   Access online forums, webinars, and caregiver support and education courses.

   o   Explore: Family Caregiver Alliance, AARP Caregiver Resource Center.

6. **Smart Home Devices**

   o   Implement voice-activated assistants and smart home technology for added convenience and safety.

   o   Consider: Amazon Alexa, Google Home, smart thermostats, and automated lighting.

Tips for Implementing Caregiving Technology:

- Start with one or two tools and gradually add more as needed.

- Ensure all caregivers are trained on how to use the technology.

- Regularly review and update your tech tools as care needs change.

- Consider the comfort level of your care recipient with technology.

Technology Type	Benefits	Considerations
Care Coordination Apps	Improved communication, task management	Requires all caregivers to adopt and use consistently
Health Monitoring Devices	Early detection of health issues, increased independence	It may require professional setup, ongoing costs
Medication Management Tools	Reduced medication errors, improved adherence	Need for regular updates, potential tech glitches
Smart Home Devices	Enhanced safety, convenience for daily tasks	Initial setup cost, learning curve for usage

Remember, effective time management and organization are ongoing processes. Be patient with yourself as you implement these strategies, and don't hesitate to adjust your approach as needed. You can create a more manageable and sustainable caregiving routine by creating a structured schedule, delegating tasks, and leveraging technology.

These tools and strategies are meant to support you, not add stress. Please choose the best methods for your unique situation and gradually incorporate them into your caregiving routine. With time and practice, you'll likely find that improved organization leads to more quality time with your loved one and better self-care for you as a caregiver.

Maintaining Personal Identity and Interests

As a caregiver, it's easy to become so immersed in your responsibilities that you lose sight of your identity and interests. However, maintaining a sense of self is crucial for your well-being and can make you a more effective caregiver. Let's explore ways to nurture your identity and interests while balancing your caregiving duties.

Pursuing Hobbies and Passions

Engaging in activities you enjoy is not a luxury—it's necessary to maintain your mental and emotional health. Here's how to keep your hobbies and passions alive:

1. **Identify Time Pockets**

   o Look for small windows of time in your schedule

   o Consider early mornings, during care recipient's naps, or after bedtime

2. **Adapt Your Hobbies**

   o Find ways to engage in your interests in shorter time frames

   o Look for portable versions of your hobbies

3. **Involve Your Care Recipient**

   o When possible, find ways to include your loved one in your activities

   o This can provide stimulation for them and enjoyment for you both

4. **Use Technology**

   o Explore online classes or virtual communities related to your interests

   o Use apps or online resources to engage in hobbies remotely

5. **Schedule Regular "Me Time"**

   o Block out time in your calendar for your interests

   o Treat this time as crucial as any other appointment

Ideas for Maintaining Hobbies:

- Reading: Join an online book club or use audiobooks during commutes

- Art: Keep a sketchbook for quick drawing sessions

- Music: Create playlists to enjoy while performing caregiving tasks

- Gardening: Start a small indoor herb garden or tend to potted plants

- Exercise: Try short workout videos or practice yoga during breaks

Hobby Type	Adaptation for Caregivers	Benefits
Reading	E-books, audiobooks, short stories	Mental stimulation, stress relief
Crafting	Portable projects (knitting, sketching)	Creativity outlet, sense of accomplishment
Fitness	Short home workouts, walking	Physical health, energy boost
Cooking	Quick recipes, meal prep	Nutrition, enjoyment, potential involvement of care recipient

Staying Connected with Friends

Maintaining social connections is vital for your emotional well-being and provides a support system outside your caregiving role. Here are strategies to stay connected:

1. **Leverage Technology**

   - Use video calls, social media, or messaging apps to stay in touch

   - Join online groups or forums related to your interests

2. **Schedule Regular Check-ins**

   o Set up recurring phone calls or virtual coffee dates with friends

   o Use calendar reminders to prompt you to reach out

3. **Be Honest About Your Situation**

   o Share your caregiving challenges with trusted friends

   o Let them know how they can support you

4. **Plan for Social Activities**

   o Arrange respite care to allow for occasional outings

   o Invite friends for short visits at home when possible

5. **Involve Friends in Caregiving**

   o Ask friends to visit or spend time with your care recipient

   o This can provide you with a break while maintaining connections

Tips for Maintaining Friendships:

- Quality over quantity: Focus on nurturing a few close relationships

- Be present: When you do have time with friends, try to be fully engaged

- Share your caregiving journey: Allow friends to understand your life

- Accept help: Let friends support you in practical ways if they offer

Connection Type	Ideas for Caregivers	Potential Challenges
Virtual Meetups	Video chat coffee dates, online game nights	Technology issues, scheduling conflicts
In-Person Visits	Short home visits, park meetups	Limited time, need for care coverage
Group Activities	Book clubs, virtual workout groups	Finding common interests, time commitment
Caregiving Involvement	Friend visits with care recipient, help with tasks	Friends' comfort level with caregiving situation

Setting Personal Goals Outside of Caregiving

Setting and working towards personal goals can provide a sense of purpose and achievement beyond your caregiving role. Here's how to approach goal-setting:

1. **Reflect on Your Aspirations**

   o   Think about what you want to achieve for yourself

   o   Consider short-term and long-term goals

2. **Start Small**

   o   Set realistic, achievable goals given your current situation

   o   Break larger goals into smaller, manageable steps

3. **Make Goals SMART**

   o   Specific, Measurable, Achievable, Relevant, Time-bound

   o   This framework helps create clear, actionable goals

4. **Write Down Your Goals**

    o   Use a journal or goal-tracking app to document your objectives

    o   Regularly review and update your goals

5. **Seek Support**

    o   Share your goals with friends or family who can encourage you

    o   Consider finding an accountability partner

6. **Celebrate Progress**

    o   Acknowledge and celebrate each step towards your goals

    o   Use achievements as motivation to continue pursuing your aspirations

Examples of Personal Goals for Caregivers:

- Learning: Take an online course or learn a new language

- Health: Establish a regular exercise routine or improve eating habits

- Career: Maintain professional skills or explore part-time work options

- Creative: Start a blog, write a book, or create art

- Personal Growth: Practice mindfulness or develop a new skill

Goal Category	Example Goal	Potential Steps
Education	Complete an online certificate program	Research programs, allocate study time, set completion date
Health and Wellness	Establish a regular meditation practice.	Download the app, start with 5 minutes daily, and gradually increase the time.
Personal Development	Improve time management skills.	Read productivity books, try a time-blocking technique, and use organization apps.
Creative Expression	Write and publish a short story	Set writing schedule, join writing group, research publishing options

Remember, maintaining your identity and interests is not selfish—it's essential for your well-being and can make you a more effective and compassionate caregiver. By pursuing your hobbies, staying connected with friends, and setting personal goals, you're taking care of yourself and bringing fresh energy and perspective to your caregiving role.

Feeling guilty about taking time for yourself is normal, but remember that self-care is crucial to sustainable caregiving—your loved one benefits when you're refreshed, fulfilled, and connected to your identity. Be patient with yourself as you navigate this balance, and don't hesitate to adjust your approach as your caregiving situation evolves. Your growth and well-being are important to you and those you care for.

Coping with Grief and Loss

As a caregiver, you may find yourself navigating complex emotions, including grief and loss, long before your loved one's passing. Understanding and addressing these feelings is crucial for your emotional well-being and ability to provide compassionate care. Let's explore how to cope with these challenging aspects of the caregiving journey.

Acknowledging Anticipatory Grief

Anticipatory grief is the grief experienced before an impending loss. For caregivers, this can begin when a loved one is diagnosed with a progressive illness or when you start to notice significant declines. Recognizing and addressing this grief is an integral part of your emotional health.

Signs of Anticipatory Grief:

- Sadness or tearfulness
- Anxiety about the future
- Loneliness or isolation
- Anger or irritability
- Guilt or regret
- Physical symptoms like fatigue or changes in appetite

Strategies for Coping with Anticipatory Grief:

1. **Acknowledge Your Feelings**
   - Recognize that your grief is valid and normal
   - Allow yourself to experience and express your emotions

2. **Seek Support**
   - Join a caregiver support group
   - Consider talking to a therapist or counselor
   - Confide in trusted friends or family members

3. **Practice Self-Care**
   - Engage in activities that bring you comfort
   - Maintain your physical health through diet and exercise
   - Set aside time for relaxation and stress relief

4. **Create Meaningful Moments**

- o Make new memories with your loved one

- o Document your journey through journaling or photography

- o Engage in life review conversations with your loved one

5. **Educate Yourself**

- o Learn about your loved one's condition and what to expect

- o Understand the grief process and its various manifestations

Emotion	Coping Strategy	Self-Care Action
Sadness	Allow yourself to cry; express emotions through art or writing	Practice gratitude journaling; spend time in nature
Anxiety	Use relaxation techniques; focus on the present moment	Try meditation or deep breathing exercises
Guilt	Challenge negative thoughts; practice self-compassion	Engage in positive self-talk; seek validation from support group
Anger	Find healthy outlets like exercise; communicate feelings assertively	Practice stress-relief techniques; consider counseling

Finding Meaning in the Caregiving Journey

While caregiving can be challenging, many find it offers opportunities for personal growth, deepened relationships, and a sense of purpose. Finding meaning in your caregiving role can help you cope with the difficulties and find moments of joy and fulfillment.

Ways to Find Meaning in Caregiving:

1. **Reflect on Your Values**

   o   Consider how caregiving aligns with your values

   o   Recognize the positive impact you're making in your loved one's life

2. **Practice Mindfulness**

   o   Stay present in the moment, appreciating small joys

   o   Use mindfulness techniques to manage stress and find peace

3. **Cultivate Gratitude**

   o   Keep a gratitude journal, noting the positive aspects of each day

   o   Share moments of appreciation with your loved one

4. **Learn and Grow**

   o   View challenges as opportunities for personal development

   o   Acquire new skills and knowledge through your caregiving role

5. **Connect with Others**

   o   Share your experiences with other caregivers

   o   Offer support and mentorship to those new to caregiving

6. **Create a Legacy Project**

   o   Work with your loved one to create something meaningful (e.g., a memory book, video, or family history project)

Find ways to honor your loved one's life and values Aspect of Caregiving	Potential for Meaning	Action to Cultivate Meaning
Daily Care Tasks	Expressing love through service	Practice mindfulness during care routines
Emotional Support	Deepening relationship bonds	Engage in life review conversations
Learning New Skills	Personal growth and empowerment	Recognize and celebrate your growing expertise
Advocating for Loved One	Standing up for what's right	Reflect on how advocacy aligns with your values

Self-Advocacy and Setting Boundaries

As a caregiver for someone with dementia, you're often so focused on your loved one's needs that you might forget to advocate for yourself. Remember, your well-being is just as important. Let's explore how you can effectively communicate your needs, set boundaries, and maintain a healthy balance in your life.

Communicating needs effectively

Effective communication is critical to meeting your needs while caring for someone with dementia. Here are some strategies to help you communicate more effectively:

1. Be clear and specific about your needs

2. Use "I" statements to express your feelings

3. Choose the right time and place for meaningful conversations

4. Practice active listening when others are speaking

5. Be open to compromise and negotiation

Communication Do's	Communication Don'ts
Express yourself calmly and respectfully.	Use accusatory language or blame others.
Be specific about what you need.	Assume others know what you're thinking.
Listen to others' perspectives.	Interrupt or dismiss others' opinions.
Take time to collect your thoughts.	React impulsively when emotions are high.

Learning to say 'no' when necessary

As a caregiver, you may feel obligated to say 'yes' to every request or task related to your loved one's care. However, learning to say 'no' when necessary is crucial for your well-being and the quality of care you provide. Here's how you can start setting limits:

- Recognize your limits: Be honest about what you can realistically handle.

- Prioritize tasks: Focus on the most essential and remove less critical responsibilities.

- Practice saying 'no': Start small and work up to more significant boundaries.

- Offer alternatives: Suggest other solutions or resources if you can't do something.

- Don't feel guilty: Remember that setting boundaries is healthy and necessary.

Balancing caregiving with other responsibilities

Striking a balance between caregiving and other aspects of your life can be challenging, but it's essential for your overall well-being. Here are some strategies to help you maintain equilibrium:

1. Create a schedule: Allocate time for caregiving, work, family, and personal activities.

2. Delegate tasks: Involve other family members or hire help for specific responsibilities.

3. Use respite care: Take advantage of short-term care options to give yourself a break.

4. Maintain your health: Prioritize your physical and mental well-being through regular check-ups and self-care.

5. Stay connected: Nurture relationships outside of your caregiving role.

Area of Life	Strategies for Balance
Work	Discuss flexible options with your employer, and consider part-time work if possible.
Family	Schedule regular family time and involve children in age-appropriate caregiving tasks.
Personal Time	Set aside time each day for activities you enjoy, even if it's just for 15 minutes.
Social Life	Join a support group and plan regular outings with friends.

Remember, caring for yourself isn't selfish—it's necessary. By advocating for your needs, setting boundaries, and maintaining balance in your life, you'll be better equipped to provide quality care for your loved one with dementia. Don't hesitate to seek support when you need it, whether from family, friends, or professional resources. You're doing important and challenging work and deserve care and support.

Continuing Education and Skills Development

As a caregiver for someone with dementia, your journey is one of continuous learning and growth. Staying informed about the latest care techniques and developing your skills can significantly improve your loved one's quality of life and your caregiving experience. Let's explore how you can enhance your knowledge and abilities in this challenging but rewarding role.

Staying informed about dementia care techniques

Dementia care is an evolving field, with new research and techniques emerging regularly. Keeping up-to-date with these developments can help you provide the best possible care for your loved one. Here are some ways to stay informed:

1. Subscribe to reputable dementia care newsletters

2. Follow leading dementia organizations on social media

3. Join online forums or support groups for caregivers

4. Read books and articles by dementia care experts

5. Consult regularly with healthcare professionals involved in your loved one's care

Resource Type	Examples	Benefits
Newsletters	Alzheimer's Association, Dementia Society of America	Regular updates on research and care techniques
Online Forums	Alzheimer's Association ALZConnected, Dementia Talking Point	Peer support and shared experiences
Books	"The 36-Hour Day" by Nancy L. Mace and Peter V. Rabins	In-depth knowledge and practical advice

Attending workshops and seminars

Workshops and seminars offer valuable opportunities to learn from experts, connect with other caregivers, and gain hands-on experience with new care techniques. Consider the following when seeking out educational opportunities:

- Look for local events hosted by hospitals, community centers, or dementia care organizations

- Explore online webinars and virtual conferences for convenient learning options

- Attend caregiver support group meetings that often feature educational components

- Investigate training programs offered by local hospice or home health agencies

- Consider certification programs in dementia care if you're looking for more comprehensive education

Remember, investing time in these educational opportunities benefits your loved one and is an act of self-care that can boost your confidence and reduce stress in your caregiving role.

Developing patience and communication skills

Caring for someone with dementia requires extraordinary patience and effective communication skills. These abilities don't always come naturally but can be developed and improved over time. Here are some strategies to enhance these crucial skills:

1. Practice mindfulness and deep breathing to stay calm in challenging situations

2. Learn about the stages of dementia to better understand and anticipate your loved one's needs

3. Use non-verbal communication techniques, such as maintaining eye contact and using a gentle touch

4. Speak clearly and slowly, using simple language and short sentences

5. Develop strategies for redirecting and de-escalating challenging behaviors

Skill	Importance	Development Strategies
Patience	Reduces stress and improves quality of care	Practice mindfulness, take regular breaks, seek support when needed
Communication	It enhances understanding and reduces frustration	Learn about non-verbal cues, practice active listening, and adjust your speaking style
Empathy	Builds trust and strengthens your relationship	Try to see situations from your loved one's perspective, and join a support group to share experiences.

Developing these skills takes time and practice. Be patient with yourself as you learn and grow in your caregiving role. Remember that every caregiver faces challenges, and it's okay to make mistakes. What's important is your commitment to learning and improving.

By staying informed about dementia care techniques, attending educational events, and continually developing your patience and communication skills, you can improve your care and take important steps to prevent burnout and maintain your well-being.

Your dedication to learning and growing as a caregiver is admirable. It reflects the depth of your commitment to your loved one and personal growth. As you continue on this journey, remember that every new skill you acquire and every bit of knowledge you gain is a valuable tool in your caregiving toolkit, helping you navigate the challenges of dementia care with greater confidence and compassion.

Planning: Legal and Financial Considerations

Taking care of a loved one with dementia is a journey that requires both compassion and preparation. As you embark on this path, addressing legal and financial matters early on is not just important; it's a responsibility. This proactive approach can save you from stress and complications, allowing you to focus on what truly matters - providing love and care for your loved one with dementia.

Understanding the Importance of Early Planning

Early planning is not just a precaution; it's a necessity. When your loved one is in the early stages of dementia, they may still have the mental capacity to make crucial decisions and express their wishes. By addressing legal and financial matters early, you:

- Ensure your loved one's voice is heard in future care decisions

- Protect their assets and finances

- Reduce potential family conflicts

- Gain peace of mind for both you and your loved one

Remember, dementia is progressive. There may come a time when your family member can no longer make sound decisions or sign legal documents. **Acting early puts you in the best position to honor their wishes and manage their care effectively.**

Financial and Legal Considerations

Navigating caregiving's financial and legal aspects can be overwhelming for a caregiver. However, understanding these elements is crucial for ensuring the best care for your loved one and protecting your financial well-being. Let's explore the key areas you need to consider.

Planning for Long-Term Care Expenses

Long-term care can be costly, and planning to manage these expenses effectively is essential. Here are some steps to help you prepare:

1. **Assess Current and Future Needs**

    o   Evaluate your loved one's current health status and potential future needs

    o   Consider the possibility of in-home care, assisted living, or nursing home care

2. **Estimate Costs**

    o   Research the costs of different care options in your area

    o   Factor in potential increases in healthcare costs over time

3. **Review Available Resources**

    o   Assess your loved one's savings, assets, and income sources

    o   Consider potential family contributions

4. **Explore Insurance Options**

    o   Look into long-term care insurance policies

    o   Understand what Medicare and Medicaid may cover

5. **Consult Financial Professionals**

    o   Speak with a financial advisor experienced in elder care planning

    o   Consider meeting with an elder law attorney

Long-Term Care Funding Options:

- Personal savings and assets

- Long-term care insurance

- Life insurance policies with long-term care riders

- Reverse mortgages (for homeowners)

- Veterans benefits (for eligible veterans and their spouses)

- Medicaid (for those who qualify based on financial need)

Care Type	Average Monthly Cost (2024)	Potential Funding Sources
In-Home Care (44 hours/week)	$4,000 - $8,000	Personal funds, LTC insurance, Medicaid waivers
Assisted Living Facility	$4,500 - $7,000	Personal funds, LTC insurance, some Medicaid programs
Nursing Home (Semi-Private Room)	$7,000 - $14,000	Medicare (short-term), Medicaid, personal funds, LTC insurance
Nursing Home (Private Room)	$8,000 - $15,000	Medicare (short-term), Medicaid, personal funds, LTC insurance
Adult Day Health Care	$1,800 - $2,600	Medicaid waivers, personal funds, some LTC insurance policies

Understanding Legal Rights and Options

Navigating the legal aspects of caregiving is crucial for protecting your loved one's interests and ensuring their wishes are respected. Here are critical legal considerations:

1. **Advance Directives**

   - Encourage your loved one to create or update their advance directives

   - Ensure you have copies of living wills and healthcare power of attorney documents

2. **Power of Attorney**

   - o Understand the difference between medical and financial power of attorney

   - o Consider setting up a durable power of attorney for finances and healthcare

3. **Guardianship/Conservatorship**

   - o Know when these might be necessary and how to pursue them if needed

   - o Understand the responsibilities and limitations of these roles

4. **Estate Planning**

   - o Encourage your loved one to create or update their will

   - o Discuss options like trusts for managing assets

5. **HIPAA Authorization**

   - o Ensure you have the necessary authorization to access your loved one's medical information

Essential Legal Documents for Caregivers:

- Durable Power of Attorney for Healthcare

- Durable Power of Attorney for Finances

- Living Will

- HIPAA Authorization Form

- Will and Trust Documents

- Do Not Resuscitate (DNR) Order (if applicable)

Legal Document	Purpose	When to Obtain
Healthcare Power of Attorney	Designates someone to make medical decisions if the person is incapacitated	As early as possible while the person can make sound decisions
Financial Power of Attorney	Allows the designated person to manage finances	Before the cognitive decline, update as needed
Living Will	Specifies end-of-life care preferences	When creating advance directives, review them periodically
HIPAA Authorization	Allows access to medical information	When beginning the caregiving role, update annually

Medical Power of Attorney: What It Is and Why It Matters

A Medical Power of Attorney (MPOA) is a legal document that allows your loved one to appoint someone they trust to make healthcare decisions on their behalf if they cannot do so themselves. This person is often called a healthcare proxy or agent.

Why is an MPOA crucial?

1. It ensures medical decisions align with your loved one's wishes

2. It prevents potential disagreements among family members about care

3. It allows for quick decision-making in emergencies

4. It gives healthcare providers a clear point of contact for meaningful discussions

To set up an MPOA:

1. Discuss the role with your loved one and decide who should be the healthcare proxy

2. Consult with an elder law attorney to draft the document

3. Ensure the document is properly signed and witnessed

4. Provide copies to healthcare providers and family members

Financial Power of Attorney: Protecting Assets and Finances

A Financial Power of Attorney (FPOA) is similar to an MPOA but focuses on financial matters. This document allows your loved one to designate someone to manage their finances if they cannot do so themselves.

Critical aspects of an FPOA:

- It can be immediate or "springing" (only taking effect under specific circumstances)

- It can be broad or limited in scope

- It ends upon the death of your loved one

Benefits of having an FPOA:

- Ensures bills are paid, and finances are managed properly

- Protects against financial exploitation

- Allows for long-term financial planning

- Provides a clear authority for financial institutions to work with

Living Wills and Advance Directives

A living will, often part of an advance directive, is a document that outlines your loved one's wishes for end-of-life care. It typically covers preferences for:

- Use of life-sustaining treatments

- Pain management and comfort care

- Organ donation

Why are these documents important?

- They provide clear guidance in difficult situations

- They reduce the emotional burden on family members making tough decisions

- They ensure your loved one's wishes are respected, even if they can't communicate

When and How to Have These Conversations

Timing is crucial when discussing these sensitive topics. Here are some tips:

1. Start early, ideally when your loved one is first diagnosed

2. Choose a calm, private setting

3. Include other family members if appropriate

4. Be patient and prepared for multiple conversations

Conversation starters:

- "I know this is hard to discuss, but I want to ensure we honor your wishes."

- "Have you thought about what kind of medical care you'd want if you couldn't make decisions?"

- "I've been reading about the importance of having certain legal documents. Can we talk about that?"

Finding Legal Assistance for Document Preparation

While finding templates for these documents online is possible, **working with an elder law attorney is highly recommended.** They can:

- Ensure documents are correctly prepared and legally binding

- Provide advice on complex family or financial situations

- Help navigate state-specific laws and requirements

To find a qualified attorney:

- Ask for recommendations from your local Alzheimer's Association chapter

- Contact your state or local bar association

- Look for attorneys certified in elder law by the National Elder Law Foundation

Proper legal preparation can save significant future stress, time, and money.

Document	Purpose	Key Points
Medical Power of Attorney	Designates someone to make healthcare decisions	• Choose a trusted individual • Discuss preferences in advance • Provide copies to healthcare providers
Financial Power of Attorney	Allows someone to manage finances	• Can be immediate or "springing" • Protects against financial exploitation • Ends upon death
Living Will/Advance Directive	Outlines end-of-life care preferences	• Covers life-sustaining treatments • Addresses pain management • Includes organ donation wishes

By addressing these legal and financial considerations early, you're taking a crucial step in ensuring the best possible care for your loved one with dementia. Remember, you're not alone in this journey. Seek support from professionals, support groups, and your community as you navigate this challenging but essential process.

Exploring Financial Assistance Programs

Various programs and resources are available to help ease the financial burden of caregiving. Here's an overview of potential assistance options:

1. **Government Programs**

   o Medicare: Understand coverage for hospital stays, doctor visits, and some home healthcare

   o Medicaid: Explore eligibility for long-term care coverage

   o Social Security Disability Insurance (SSDI): For those under 65 with qualifying disabilities

   o Supplemental Security Income (SSI): For low-income individuals with disabilities

2. **Veterans Benefits**

   o Aid and Attendance benefits for veterans and surviving spouses

   o Veteran-Directed Care Program

   o VA Caregiver Support Program

3. **State and Local Programs**

   o Area Agencies on Aging: Local resources and support programs

   o State-specific caregiver support programs

   o Respite care grants or vouchers

4. **Non-Profit Organizations**

   o Disease-specific organizations offering financial assistance

   o Local charities and community organizations

5. **Employer Benefits**

   - o   Check if your employer offers caregiver support or flexible work arrangements

   - o   Employee Assistance Programs (EAPs) may provide counseling or referrals

6. **Tax Deductions and Credits**

   - o   Explore potential tax benefits for caregivers

   - o   Consult a tax professional to understand your eligibility

Steps to Access Financial Assistance:

1. Research programs you might be eligible for

2. Gather necessary documentation (medical records, financial information)

3. Contact program administrators or local offices for application procedures

4. Consider seeking help from a social worker or case manager to navigate options

5. Be persistent and don't hesitate to appeal if initially denied

Assistance Type	Potential Programs	Eligibility Factors
Government Assistance	Medicare, Medicaid, SSDI, SSI	Age, disability status, income, assets
Veterans Benefits	Aid and Attendance, VA Caregiver Support	Military service, disability rating, income
State Programs	Caregiver support, respite care grants	Varies by state, often based on need
Non-Profit Assistance	Disease-specific org grants, local charities	Diagnosis, financial need, location

Remember, navigating caregiving's financial and legal aspects can be complex, but you don't have to do it alone. Don't hesitate to seek professional advice from financial advisors, elder law attorneys, or social workers specializing in senior care. Many communities offer free or low-cost legal clinics and financial counseling services for caregivers.

Addressing these matters early and revisiting them regularly as circumstances change is essential. By understanding and planning for caregiving's financial and legal aspects, you can ensure better care for your loved one and protect your financial well-being.

Understanding and managing these considerations can provide peace of mind, allowing you to focus more energy on the day-to-day aspects of caregiving and your relationship with your loved one. Remember, being proactive in these areas is an integral part of your role as a caregiver and a vital aspect of self-care.

Validation Therapy

Naomi Feil's Validation Therapy

Validation Therapy is a compassionate approach developed by Naomi Feil to help people with dementia feel understood and valued. It involves acknowledging and validating their feelings and experiences rather than trying to correct or dismiss them.

History and Development

Naomi Feil, a social worker, developed validation therapy between 1963 and 1980. She grew up in a family home for seniors and noticed that traditional therapies often upset or isolated elderly patients with dementia. She sought a better way to communicate with them, leading to the creation of Validation Therapy.

Key milestones:

- **1963-1980:** Development of Validation Therapy by Naomi Feil

- **1982:** Publication of Feil's first book on Validation Therapy

- **1980s:** Gained attention in the U.S. through presentations and research

Core Principles

Validation Therapy is based on several core principles guiding caregivers' interactions with dementia patients.

Core principles include:

1. **Acceptance:** Accept the person where they are and where they are not.

2. **Empathy:** Step into their world and feel what they feel.

3. **Respect:** Validate their emotions and experiences without judgment.

4. **Communication:** Use verbal and non-verbal techniques to connect.

Principle	Description
Acceptance	Accept the person as they are
Empathy	Feel what they feel.
Respect	Validate emotions and experiences.
Communication	Use verbal and non-verbal techniques.

Benefits for Dementia Patients

Validation Therapy offers numerous benefits for dementia patients, helping them feel more connected and less isolated.

Benefits include:

- **Restoration of self-worth:** Patients feel valued and understood.

- **Reduced withdrawal:** Encourages interaction with others.

- **Decreased stress and anxiety:** Provides emotional comfort.

- **Improved communication:** Enhances the ability to express feelings.

- **Stimulation of potential:** Helps patients engage in meaningful activities.

Benefit	Description
Restoration of self-worth	Patients feel valued and understood.
Reduced withdrawal	Encourages interaction with others
Decreased stress and anxiety	Provides emotional comfort
Improved communication	Enhances ability to express feelings
Stimulation of potential	Helps patients engage in meaningful activities

Techniques and Examples

Validation Therapy uses specific techniques to connect with dementia patients and validate their feelings.

Techniques include:

- **Mirroring:** Reflecting the patient's body language and emotions.

- **Rephrasing:** Restating what the patient says to show understanding.

- **Reminiscence:** Encouraging patients to talk about past experiences.

- **Touch:** Using gentle touch to convey empathy and support.

- **Eye contact:** Maintaining eye contact to build trust.

Examples of techniques:

1. **Mirroring:**

   - If a patient is wringing their hands, the caregiver might gently mimic this action to show empathy.

2. **Rephrasing:**

   - Patient: "I need to find my mother."

   - Caregiver: "You miss your mother and want to see her."

3. **Reminiscence:**

   - Asking the patient about their favorite childhood memory.

4. **Touch:**

   - Holding the patient's hand during a conversation.

5. **Eye contact:**

   - Looking into the patient's eyes while speaking to them.

Technique	Example
Mirroring	Mimicking hand-wringing to show empathy
Rephrasing	"You miss your mother and want to see her."
Reminiscence	Asking about favorite childhood memory
Touch	Holding the patient's hand
Eye contact	Maintaining eye contact during conversation

Using these techniques, caregivers can create a supportive and understanding environment for dementia patients, helping them feel more secure and less anxious. Validation Therapy is a powerful tool that respects the dignity and emotions of those with dementia, fostering meaningful connections and improving their overall well-being.

Other Validation Techniques

In addition to Naomi Feil's Validation Therapy, several other nonpharmacological methods can be effective in managing dementia symptoms. These methods focus on empathetic communication and creating a supportive environment for dementia patients.

Empathetic Listening

Empathetic listening involves genuinely hearing and understanding what the person with dementia is saying verbally and non-verbally.

Steps for empathetic listening:

1. **Be present:** Give your full attention to the person.

2. **Acknowledge feelings:** Reflect on what you hear to show understanding.

3. **Avoid judgment:** Accept their feelings without trying to correct them.

4. **Use non-verbal cues:** Nod, maintain eye contact, and use appropriate facial expressions.

Example:

- Patient: "I feel so lost."

- Caregiver: "It sounds like you're feeling confused and scared. I'm here with you."

Reassurance and Comfort

Providing reassurance and comfort can help alleviate fear and anxiety in dementia patients.

Ways to provide reassurance:

- **Verbal reassurance:** Use calming and soothing words.

- **Physical comfort:** Offer a gentle touch or a hug.

- **Familiar objects:** Provide comfort items, like a favorite blanket or photo.

Example:

- Patient: "I can't find my way home."

- Caregiver: "You're safe here with me. Let's sit together and talk."

Reminiscence Therapy

Reminiscence therapy involves encouraging dementia patients to talk about their past experiences. This can help them feel more connected and valued.

Benefits of reminiscence therapy:

- **Improves mood:** Talking about happy memories can boost spirits.

- **Enhances communication:** Encourages verbal expression.

- **Strengthens identity:** Helps patients remember who they are.

Techniques for reminiscence therapy:

- **Use photos:** Show old family photos and ask about the people and events in them.

- **Music:** Play songs from their youth and discuss memories associated with the music.

- **Objects:** Use familiar objects to trigger memories and conversations.

Example:

- Caregiver: "Do you remember this photo from your wedding day? Tell me about that day."

Reality Orientation

Reality orientation involves gently reminding dementia patients of the current time, place, and situation to help reduce confusion.

Techniques for reality orientation:

- **Use calendars and clocks:** Place them in visible locations.

- **Daily routines:** Maintain consistent daily schedules.

- **Verbal reminders:** Gently remind them of the date, time, and location.

Example:

- Caregiver: "Good morning, it's Tuesday, June 22nd. We're at home, and it's time for breakfast."

Distraction and Redirection

Distraction and redirection involve shifting the patient's focus from distressing thoughts or behaviors to something more positive.

Techniques for distraction and redirection:

- **Engage in activities:** Suggest a favorite hobby or task.

- **Change the environment:** Move to a different room or walk.

- **Use humor:** Light-hearted jokes or funny stories can help.

Example:

- Patient: "I need to go to work."

- Caregiver: "Let's take a walk in the garden first. Look at these beautiful flowers!"

Cognitive Stimulation Therapy

Cognitive Stimulation Therapy (CST) involves engaging dementia patients in activities that stimulate thinking and memory.

Benefits of CST:

- **Improves cognitive function:** Helps maintain mental abilities.

- **Enhances social interaction:** Encourages group activities and communication.

- **Boosts mood:** Engaging in activities can reduce depression and anxiety.

Examples of CST activities:

- **Puzzles and games:** Crosswords, Sudoku, and memory games.

- **Arts and crafts:** Painting, drawing, and crafting.

- **Group discussions:** Talking about current events or shared interests.

Example:

- Caregiver: "Let's work on this puzzle together. Can you find the corner pieces?"

Environmental Modifications

Modifying the environment can help reduce confusion and agitation in dementia patients.

Tips for environmental modifications:

- **Simplify the space:** Remove clutter and unnecessary items.

- **Use clear signage:** Label rooms and essential items.

- **Ensure safety:** Install grab bars, remove tripping hazards, and use nightlights.

Example:

- Caregiver: "I've labeled the bathroom door and put a nightlight in the hallway to help you find your way at night."

Technique	Description	Example
Empathetic Listening	Genuinely hearing and understanding the patient	"It sounds like you're feeling confused and scared. I'm here with you."
Reassurance and Comfort	Providing verbal and physical comfort	"You're safe here with me. Let's sit together and talk."
Reminiscence Therapy	Encouraging talk about past experiences	"Do you remember this photo from your wedding day? Tell me about that day."
Reality Orientation	Gently reminding of the current time, place, and situation	"Good morning, it's Tuesday, June 22nd. We're at home, and it's time for breakfast."
Distraction and Redirection	Shifting the focus to something positive	"Let's take a walk in the garden first. Look at these beautiful flowers!"
Cognitive Stimulation Therapy	Engaging in activities that stimulate thinking	"Let's work on this puzzle together. Can you find the corner pieces?"
Environmental Modifications	Modifying the environment to reduce confusion	"I've labeled the bathroom door and put a nightlight in the hallway to help you find your way at night."

By using these nonpharmacological methods, caregivers can create a supportive and understanding environment for dementia patients, helping them feel more secure and less anxious. These techniques respect the dignity and emotions of those with dementia, fostering meaningful connections and improving their overall well-being.

Practical Strategies for Caregivers

Caring for someone with dementia can be challenging, but with the right strategies, you can significantly improve their quality of life. Let's explore some practical approaches to help you provide the best care possible.

Identifying and Addressing Unmet Needs

People with dementia may struggle to communicate their needs, leading to frustration and behavioral issues. You can often prevent or reduce challenging behaviors by identifying and addressing these unmet needs.

Common unmet needs to look out for:

- Physical discomfort (pain, hunger, thirst)

- Emotional distress (loneliness, boredom, anxiety)

- Environmental factors (too hot, too cold, too noisy)

- Need for routine or structure

Steps to identify and address unmet needs:

1. **Observe closely:** Watch for changes in behavior or mood.

2. **Keep a log:** Note patterns in behavior and potential triggers.

3. **Check for physical discomfort:** Ensure basic needs (food, water, toileting) are met.

4. **Offer comfort:** Provide reassurance and emotional support.

5. **Adjust the environment:** Make changes to reduce stress or discomfort.

Need	Possible Signs	Potential Solutions
Hunger/Thirst	Agitation, wandering	Offer snacks or drinks regularly
Pain	Grimacing, guarding a body part	Consult with a doctor for pain management
Boredom	Restlessness, repetitive behaviors	Engage in meaningful activities
Overstimulation	Agitation, trying to leave	Create a calm, quiet space

Creating a Safe and Stable Environment

A safe and stable environment can significantly reduce anxiety and confusion for someone with dementia.

Tips for creating a safe environment:

- **Remove hazards:** Clear clutter, secure loose rugs, and remove dangerous items.

- **Enhance visibility:** Use contrasting colors for essential objects and improve lighting.

- **Simplify the space:** Reduce unnecessary furniture and decorations.

- **Use labels:** Clearly label essential rooms and items.

- **Maintain consistency:** Keep furniture arrangements stable and routines predictable.

Creating a dementia-friendly home:

1. **Kitchen:** Lock up hazardous items and use appliances with automatic shut-off features.

2. **Bathroom:** Install grab bars, use non-slip mats, and consider a raised toilet seat.

3. **Bedroom:** Ensure a clear path to the bathroom, and use nightlights.

4. **Living areas:** Remove or secure items that could cause trips or falls.

Communication Tips for De-escalating Fear

Effective communication is critical to managing fear and anxiety in someone with dementia.

General communication tips:

- Speak clearly and slowly

- Use simple language and short sentences

- Maintain eye contact and a calm demeanor

- Use a gentle touch when appropriate

Strategies for de-escalating fear:

1. **Validate feelings:** Acknowledge their emotions without judgment.

   - Example: "I can see you're feeling scared. It's okay, I'm here with you."

2. **Use distraction:** Redirect attention to a pleasant topic or activity.

   - Example: "Let's look at your family photo album together."

3. **Provide reassurance:** Offer comfort and support.

   - Example: "You're safe here. I'll stay with you until you feel better."

4. **Create a calm environment:** Reduce noise and distractions.

   - Example: Turn off the TV, close curtains, or move to a quieter room.

5. **Use visual cues:** Show, don't just tell.

   - Example: If it's time for a meal, show them the table set with food.

De-escalation techniques:

Technique	Description	Example
Validation	Acknowledge feelings	"I understand you're feeling upset."
Distraction	Redirect attention	"Would you like to help me fold these towels?"
Reassurance	Provide comfort	"You're safe here with me."
Environment	Create calm	Reduce noise, adjust lighting
Visual cues	Show, don't tell	Point to or show objects instead of just describing them

Remember, every person with dementia is unique, and what works for one may not work for another. Be patient, flexible, and willing to try different approaches. Your compassion and understanding can make a world of difference in the life of someone with dementia.

Case Studies and Real-Life Examples

Understanding how different approaches work in real-life situations can be incredibly helpful for caregivers. Here, we will explore success stories with Validation Therapy and how combining pharmacological and nonpharmacological approaches can be effective.

Success Stories with Validation Therapy

Validation Therapy has been used successfully in many cases to improve the quality of life for dementia patients. Here are a few examples:

Case Study 1: Mrs. Johnson

Background:

- Mrs. Johnson, an 85-year-old woman with Alzheimer's disease, frequently called out for her deceased mother, causing distress to herself and her caregivers.

Approach:

- Caregivers used Validation Therapy by acknowledging her feelings and gently engaging her in conversations about her mother.

Outcome:

- Mrs. Johnson became calmer and more content. She started sharing happy memories about her mother, which reduced her anxiety and agitation.

Case Study 2: Mr. Smith

Background:

- Mr. Smith, a 78-year-old man with Lewy body dementia, often saw imaginary animals in his room, leading to fear and confusion.

Approach:

- Caregivers used Validation Therapy by acknowledging his fear and gently redirecting his attention to a favorite activity, like listening to music.

- Mr. Smith's episodes of fear decreased, and he became more engaged in activities he enjoyed, improving his overall mood.

Case Study	Background	Approach	Outcome
Mrs. Johnson	Called out for deceased mother	Acknowledged feelings, engaged in conversations about mother	Reduced anxiety and agitation
Mr. Smith	Saw imaginary animals	Acknowledged fear, redirected to a favorite activity	Decreased fear, improved mood

By using these nonpharmacological methods, caregivers can create a supportive and understanding environment for dementia patients, helping them feel more secure and less anxious. These techniques respect the dignity and emotions of those with dementia, fostering meaningful connections and improving their overall well-being.

CPAP

Caring for a loved one with dementia can be incredibly rewarding but also challenging, especially when it comes to ensuring they use medical devices like a CPAP machine. CPAP, or Continuous Positive Airway Pressure, is essential for individuals with sleep apnea to breathe easily and sleep well through the night. However, getting someone with dementia to wear a CPAP overnight can be difficult. This article will provide practical tips and strategies to help you manage this task, ensuring your loved one gets the best care possible.

Understanding the Challenge

Helping a person with dementia use a CPAP machine overnight can be challenging for several reasons:

1. **Cognitive Impairment:** Dementia affects memory, reasoning, and the ability to understand new information, making it hard for people with dementia to remember why they need to wear the CPAP mask.

2. **Anxiety and Fear:** The CPAP machine and mask can seem strange and scary to someone with dementia. They might not understand what it is or why it's necessary.

3. **Physical Discomfort:** Wearing the CPAP mask can be uncomfortable, and adjusting to the sensation of the air pressure can be difficult, especially for someone with cognitive impairment.

4. **Restlessness:** Many people with dementia experience restlessness or agitation, which can lead them to remove the CPAP mask during the night.

Importance of CPAP Therapy for Dementia Patients

Using a CPAP machine correctly is crucial for individuals with sleep apnea, including those with dementia. Here's why:

1. **Improves Sleep Quality:** CPAP therapy helps keep the airway open, preventing pauses in breathing that disrupt sleep. Better

sleep can improve overall mood and cognitive function in dementia patients.

2. **Prevents Health Complications:** Untreated sleep apnea can lead to serious health problems such as high blood pressure, heart disease, and stroke. By ensuring your loved one uses their CPAP machine, you're helping protect their long-term health.

3. **Enhances Daytime Alertness:** Poor sleep can lead to excessive daytime sleepiness and confusion, worsening dementia symptoms. Using CPAP can help your loved one feel more awake and alert during the day.

4. **Reduces Nocturnal Disturbances:** Proper use of CPAP can reduce nighttime awakenings, leading to more restful nights for both the patient and the caregiver.

Preparation Before Bedtime

Ensuring that your loved one with dementia uses their CPAP machine effectively starts with good preparation before bedtime. A few simple steps can significantly affect how smoothly things go. Here are some key strategies to help you prepare:

Create a Calm Environment

Creating a calm and peaceful environment is crucial for helping your loved one feel comfortable and less anxious before bedtime. Here are some tips:

1. **Reduce Noise and Light:** Turn off loud appliances and dim the lights in the bedroom to create a quiet and soothing atmosphere. Soft, calming music can also help.

2. **Comfortable Temperature:** Ensure the room is not too hot or cold. This will help your loved one relax and get ready for sleep.

3. **Soothing Scents:** Consider using calming scents like lavender or chamomile. You can use an essential oil diffuser or lightly spray a lavender scent on the pillow.

4. **Familiar Items:** Surround your loved one with familiar and comforting items such as a favorite blanket or stuffed animal. Familiar objects can provide a sense of security and ease anxiety.

Establish a Bedtime Routine

A consistent bedtime routine can help signal your loved one that it's time to wind down and get ready for sleep. Routines benefit people with dementia by creating a sense of predictability and security. Here's how to establish one:

1. **Consistent Bedtime:** Try to put your loved one to bed simultaneously every night. Consistency helps regulate their internal clock and improves sleep quality.

2. **Relaxing Activities:** Before bed, engage in calming activities such as reading a book, listening to soothing music, or taking a warm bath. Avoid stimulating activities like watching TV or using a computer.

3. **Simple Steps:** Break the bedtime routine into simple, easy-to-follow steps. For example, brush teeth, change into pajamas, read a story, and then put on the CPAP mask. Keep the steps the same each night.

4. **Positive Reinforcement:** Praise and encourage your loved one throughout the routine. Positive reinforcement can help them feel more cooperative and willing to follow the routine.

Familiarize with CPAP Equipment

Helping your loved one get used to the CPAP equipment can reduce their anxiety and increase their willingness to use it. Here are some ways to familiarize them with the equipment:

1. **Show and Explain:** When your loved one is calm during the day, show them the CPAP machine and mask and explain how it helps them breathe better at night.

2. **Practice Time:** Allow them to touch and handle the mask and machine. Let them practice wearing the mask for short periods during the day to get used to how it feels.

3. **Gradual Introduction:** If your loved one is anxious, introduce the CPAP mask gradually. Start by just holding it near their face, then progress to wearing it loosely, and finally secure it properly.

4. **Model the Behavior:** Demonstrate how to wear the mask yourself or have another family member do it. Seeing someone else use the CPAP can make it seem less intimidating.

5. **Make it Comfortable:** Ensure the mask is appropriately adjusted to fit comfortably. A well-fitting mask is less likely to be bothersome and more likely to stay on throughout the night.

By creating a calm environment, establishing a consistent bedtime routine, and helping your loved one get comfortable with the CPAP equipment, you can significantly improve their willingness and ability to use the CPAP machine effectively. These preparations can make bedtime smoother and more restful for you and your loved one.

Tips for Successful CPAP Use

Helping a dementia patient use a CPAP machine successfully involves several strategies. These tips focus on making the CPAP experience as comfortable and practical as possible. By addressing key aspects such as mask choice, fit, and machine settings, you can significantly enhance your loved one's willingness to use the device consistently.

Choosing the Right CPAP Mask

Selecting a suitable CPAP mask is crucial for comfort and effectiveness. There are different types of masks, and choosing one that suits your loved one's needs can make a big difference:

1. **Types of Masks:**

   - **Nasal Masks:** Cover the nose only. Suitable for people who breathe through their nose.

   - **Full-Face Masks:** Cover both the nose and mouth. Ideal for mouth-breathers or those with nasal congestion.

   - **Nasal Pillow Masks:** These rest at the entrance of the nostrils. They are less intrusive and suitable for those who feel claustrophobic.

2. **Comfort and Preferences:**

   - **Soft Padding:** Look for masks with soft padding to reduce pressure on the face.

o **Lightweight Design:** A lighter mask can be more comfortable and less intimidating.

3. **Trial and Error:**

   o **Try Different Masks:** It might take a few different masks to find the one your loved one finds most comfortable. Don't be afraid to experiment.

   o **Consult a Specialist:** Work with a healthcare provider or a CPAP specialist to get recommendations and fittings.

Ensuring Proper Mask Fit

A properly fitting mask is essential for effective CPAP therapy. An ill-fitting mask can cause discomfort and leaks, which can make the treatment less effective and more frustrating:

1. **Proper Fit:**

   o **Adjustable Straps:** Make sure the mask has adjustable straps to customize the fit.

   o **No Gaps:** Ensure no gaps between the mask and the skin to prevent air leaks.

2. **Comfort Checks:**

   o **Skin Comfort:** Check that the mask is not causing any red marks or pressure sores.

   o **No Tightness:** The mask should be snug but not too tight. Over-tightening can cause discomfort and skin irritation.

3. **Regular Adjustments:**

   o **Check Every Night:** Adjust the mask before bedtime to ensure it fits well.

   o **Listen to Complaints:** Respond to any complaints your loved one might have about the mask and adjust as needed.

Adjusting CPAP Settings for Comfort

The CPAP machine settings can be adjusted to improve comfort, making it more likely that your loved one will use it consistently:

1. **Pressure Settings:**

     o **Start Low:** Start with a lower pressure setting and gradually increase it to the prescribed level. This can help your loved one get used to the sensation.

     o **Auto-Adjusting Machines:** Some CPAP machines can automatically adjust the pressure throughout the night based on your loved one's breathing patterns. This can enhance comfort.

2. **Ramp Feature:**

     o **Gradual Increase:** Use the CPAP machine's ramp feature, which starts at a lower pressure and gradually increases to the prescribed level. This can help your loved one fall asleep more comfortably.

3. **Humidification:**

     o **Add a Humidifier:** CPAP machines often have a humidification feature to add moisture to the air, which can prevent dryness in the nose and throat.

     o **Adjust Humidity Levels:** Experiment with the humidity levels to find the most comfortable setting for your loved one.

4. **Noise Levels:**

     o **Quiet Machines:** Ensure the CPAP machine is as quiet as possible. Older machines can be noisy and disruptive.

     o **Positioning:** Place the machine on a stable surface and use soft padding underneath it to reduce vibrations and noise.

5. **Comfort Settings:**

   o **Flex Settings:** Some CPAP machines offer settings that reduce pressure during exhalation, making it easier to breathe out against the air pressure.

Ensuring successful CPAP use for a loved one with dementia involves careful consideration of mask choice, fit, and machine settings. By choosing a comfortable mask, providing it fits properly, and adjusting the CPAP settings to enhance comfort, you can help your loved one use their CPAP machine more consistently and effectively. These efforts can improve their sleep quality, overall health, and well-being, significantly impacting their life and yours.

Behavioral Strategies

Helping a loved one with dementia use their CPAP machine successfully often requires more than just the right equipment and settings. Behavioral strategies can play a significant role in encouraging cooperation and ensuring the CPAP machine is used consistently. Here are some practical approaches:

Positive Reinforcement and Encouragement

Positive reinforcement can be a powerful tool in encouraging your loved one to use their CPAP machine. Here's how to use it effectively:

1. **Praise and Compliments:**

   o **Acknowledge Effort:** Praise your loved one whenever they try to use the CPAP machine, even if they don't use it ideally. Recognize their effort and cooperation.

   o **Specific Compliments:** Be specific about what they did well. For example, "You did a great job keeping the mask on tonight!"

2. **Rewards:**

   o **Small Rewards:** Offer small rewards for using the CPAP machine, such as a favorite snack, a particular activity, or extra time doing something they enjoy.

o **Incentive Chart:** Use an incentive chart to track successful nights with the CPAP. Small rewards can be given for meeting goals, such as keeping the mask on for hours.

3. **Positive Language:**

   o **Encouraging Words:** Use positive and encouraging language. Instead of saying, "You have to wear this," try saying, "This will help you breathe easier and feel better."

4. **Celebrate Successes:**

   o **Celebrate Achievements:** Celebrate small victories. For example, if your loved one keeps the mask on longer than usual, acknowledge this achievement enthusiastically.

Distraction Techniques

Distraction techniques can help divert your loved one's attention away from the CPAP machine and reduce anxiety or resistance. Here are some methods:

1. **Engaging Activities:**

   o **Favorite Activities:** Before bed, engage your loved one in a favorite activity to help them relax. This could be reading a book, listening to music, or watching a favorite show.

   o **Games and Puzzles:** Simple games or puzzles can keep their mind occupied and distract them from any discomfort associated with the CPAP mask.

2. **Sensory Distractions:**

   o **Soft Music:** Play soft, calming music or nature sounds in the background while putting on the CPAP mask.

   o **Aromatherapy:** Use pleasant scents like lavender or chamomile to create a relaxing environment and distract from the mask.

3. **Engage in Conversation:**

- o **Talk About Positive Topics:** While wearing the mask, engage in light, positive conversation. Talking about happy memories or upcoming events can shift focus away from the CPAP machine.

4. **Bedtime Stories:**

- o **Read Aloud:** Read a favorite book or tell a comforting story as your loved one settles into bed with the CPAP mask. The familiar and enjoyable activity can provide comfort and distraction.

Consistency and Patience

Consistency and patience are key when helping a loved one with dementia use their CPAP machine. Here's how to apply these principles effectively:

1. **Establish Routine:**

- o **Same Time Every Night:** Put on the CPAP mask simultaneously every night to create a sense of routine and predictability.

- o **Consistent Steps:** Follow the same steps every night when preparing for bed and wearing the mask. Repetition can help your loved one feel more comfortable and secure.

2. **Be Patient:**

- o **Stay Calm:** Remain calm and patient, even if your loved one resists or gets frustrated. Your calm demeanor can help reduce their anxiety.

- o **Take Breaks:** If your loved one becomes very upset, take a short break and try again in a few minutes. Pushing too hard can increase resistance.

3. **Gradual Process:**

   o **Start Slow:** Introduce the CPAP mask gradually. Start with short periods during the day and slowly increase the time as your loved one becomes more comfortable.

   o **Celebrate Progress:** Celebrate each small step of progress, no matter how minor. Recognize that adapting to the CPAP machine is a gradual process.

4. **Involve Them in the Process:**

   o **Seek Input:** Involve your loved one in the process as much as possible. Ask them how the mask feels and if they need any adjustments to be more comfortable.

   o **Empowerment:** Empower them by giving them some control, like choosing when to start the bedtime routine or selecting a favorite calming activity.

Behavioral strategies such as positive reinforcement, distraction techniques, consistency, and patience can significantly enhance your loved one's willingness to use their CPAP machine. These approaches can make the experience more positive and manageable for you and your loved one. By understanding and implementing these strategies, you're helping them with their CPAP therapy and showing empathy, patience, and support in their care journey.

Handling Resistance

It's common for individuals with dementia to resist using medical equipment like a CPAP machine. This resistance can stem from various factors, and handling it requires a gentle and understanding approach. Here are strategies to identify resistance causes, gently redirection techniques, and consult healthcare providers for solutions.

Identifying Causes of Resistance

Understanding why your loved one resists using their CPAP machine is the first step in addressing the issue. Here are some common causes:

1. **Fear and Anxiety:**

    o   **Unfamiliarity:** The CPAP mask and machine can seem strange and intimidating. Your loved one might not understand what it is or why they need it.

    o   **Fear of Suffocation:** Some people may feel claustrophobic or fear the mask will suffocate them.

2. **Discomfort:**

    o   **Physical Discomfort:** The mask might be uncomfortable or cause skin irritation. The pressure from the machine can also feel unnatural or bothersome.

    o   **Dryness:** CPAP therapy can cause dryness in the nose and throat, leading to discomfort.

3. **Cognitive Impairment:**

    o   **Memory Issues:** Your loved one might forget why they must wear the CPAP mask or how to use it.

    o   **Confusion:** Dementia can confuse and make it difficult for them to understand instructions or the importance of the device.

4. **Restlessness and Agitation:**

    o   **Restless Behavior:** People with dementia often experience restlessness or agitation, especially in the evening. This can make it challenging to keep the mask on.

Gentle Redirection Techniques

When your loved one resists using the CPAP machine, gentle redirection techniques can help guide them back to using it without causing further distress. Here are some methods:

1. **Calm and Reassuring Communication:**

    o **Stay Calm:** Keep your voice calm and reassuring. Speak slowly and use simple language to explain why the CPAP machine is essential.

    o **Positive Tone:** Use a positive and encouraging tone. Avoid showing frustration or anger, as this can increase resistance.

2. **Distraction:**

    o **Engage in Activities:** Distract your loved one with a favorite activity or calming task. For example, you might play soft music, read a book, or engage in light conversation.

    o **Focus on the Positive:** Talk about something they enjoy or look forward to. Redirecting their attention to something pleasant can reduce anxiety.

3. **Step-by-Step Guidance:**

    o **Break It Down:** Break down the process into small, manageable steps. Guide your loved one through each step slowly and patiently.

    o **Use Visual Cues:** Demonstrate how to put on the mask or show pictures of others using it. Visual cues can help them understand better.

4. **Comfort and Security:**

    o **Reassure Them:** Offer reassurance and comfort. Hold their hand or give a gentle touch to make them feel secure.

    o **Create a Cozy Environment:** Make the bedroom as cozy and inviting as possible. A comfortable environment can help reduce resistance.

Consulting Healthcare Providers for Solutions

When all your efforts fail to overcome resistance, seeking help from healthcare providers is crucial. They can provide professional advice and tailored solutions to address your loved one's needs:

1. **CPAP Specialists:**

   o **Expert Advice:** Consult a CPAP specialist for guidance on mask fitting, pressure settings, and other adjustments to improve comfort.

   o **Equipment Options:** They might suggest different types of masks or machines that could be more suitable for your loved one.

2. **Medical Professionals:**

   o **Doctor's Input:** Talk to your loved one's doctor about the resistance. They can check for any medical issues causing discomfort, such as nasal congestion or skin irritation.

   o **Medication Review:** The doctor can review medications to ensure no side effects contribute to restlessness or agitation.

3. **Behavioral Therapists:**

   o **Therapeutic Techniques:** A behavioral therapist can work with your loved one to address anxiety, fear, and other emotional issues related to using the CPAP machine.

   o **Tailored Strategies:** They can develop personalized strategies to help your loved one feel more comfortable and cooperative.

4. **Support Groups:**

   o **Caregiver Support:** Join support groups for caregivers of individuals with dementia. Sharing experiences and solutions with others in similar situations can provide new insights and encouragement.

   o **Patient Support:** Some groups offer direct patient support, including advice on managing medical devices like CPAP machines.

Handling resistance to CPAP therapy in loved ones with dementia involves identifying the underlying causes, using gentle redirection techniques, and consulting healthcare providers for solutions. You can help your loved one use their CPAP machine more effectively and comfortably by approaching the situation with empathy, patience, and professional support. This improves their health and well-being and creates a more peaceful and positive caregiving experience.

Monitoring and Adjusting

Ensuring that your loved one with dementia successfully uses their CPAP machine requires ongoing monitoring and adjustments. This continuous care approach helps address any issues promptly, providing the therapy remains practical and comfortable. Here are some strategies for monitoring and adjusting CPAP use.

Regular Check-ins

Regular check-ins are essential to ensure the CPAP therapy works well and identify problems early on. Here's how to conduct effective check-ins:

1. **Daily Observations:**

   o **Visual Checks:** Check if the mask was correctly worn overnight each morning. Look for any signs of discomfort, such as red marks or pressure sores on the face.

- o **Behavioral Signs:** Observe your loved one's behavior and mood. Are they more rested, less irritable, or more alert during the day? Positive changes can indicate the therapy is working well.

2. **Comfort Assessments:**

   - o **Ask for Feedback:** Gently ask your loved one how they felt using the CPAP machine. They might express discomfort, even if they can't articulate it well. Look for non-verbal cues, like touching or rubbing the face.

   - o **Check for Issues:** Regularly check for mask leaks, dryness, or nasal congestion. These can affect the effectiveness of the CPAP therapy and your loved one's comfort.

3. **Tracking Progress:**

   - o **Keep a Journal:** Maintain a journal to track nightly use, any issues observed, and how your loved one feels daily. This can help you identify patterns and make informed adjustments.

   - o **Monitor Sleep Quality:** Pay attention to sleep quality indicators like fewer nighttime awakenings and less daytime sleepiness, which suggest the therapy is effective.

Adjusting Strategies as Needed

Based on your observations and check-ins, you might need to adjust strategies to ensure continued success with CPAP therapy. Here's how to make those adjustments:

1. **Mask Adjustments:**

   - o **Fit and Comfort:** Adjust the straps for a better fit if the mask seems uncomfortable. Make sure it's snug but not too tight. A comfortable mask is more likely to stay on all night.

   - o **Type of Mask:** If discomfort persists, try a different mask. For example, a nasal pillow mask might be more comfortable than a full-face mask.

2. **Pressure Settings:**

   o **Review Settings:** If your loved one struggles with air pressure, consult a healthcare provider to review and adjust the settings. Sometimes, starting with a lower pressure and gradually increasing it can help.

   o **Ramp Feature:** Use the CPAP machine's ramp feature, which starts the pressure low and gradually increases it, making it easier for your loved one to fall asleep.

3. **Environmental Adjustments:**

   o **Room Conditions:** Ensure the room is quiet, dark, and cool, which can help your loved one sleep better with the CPAP machine.

   o **Humidification:** If dryness is an issue, adjust the humidification settings on the CPAP machine to add more moisture to the air.

4. **Routine Adjustments:**

   o **Bedtime Routine:** Re-evaluate and adjust the bedtime routine if needed. Sometimes, slight changes, like introducing a calming activity or adjusting the timing, can improve cooperation.

Involving Professional Support

Sometimes, despite your best efforts, additional professional support is needed to ensure the CPAP therapy is successful. Here's how to involve professionals:

1. **Healthcare Providers:**

   o **Regular Check-ups:** Schedule regular check-ups with your loved one's doctor to review the effectiveness of the CPAP therapy and address any medical concerns.

   o **Sleep Specialists:** Consult a sleep specialist who can provide in-depth analysis and adjustments to the CPAP machine and therapy plan.

2. **CPAP Technicians:**

   o **Technical Support:** Work with CPAP technicians who can help troubleshoot and resolve any technical issues with the machine or mask.

   o **Equipment Upgrades:** They can also suggest and provide newer or different equipment that might be more comfortable or effective.

3. **Behavioral Therapists:**

   o **Therapy Sessions:** Engage a behavioral therapist to help manage any anxiety or behavioral issues related to using the CPAP machine. They can teach coping strategies and provide support.

   o **Personalized Strategies:** Therapists can develop personalized strategies to address resistance and improve cooperation.

4. **Support Groups:**

   o **Caregiver Support:** Join caregiver support groups where you can share experiences and get advice from others facing similar challenges. These groups can offer practical tips and emotional support.

   o **Patient Support:** Some support groups also cater directly to patients, offering activities and advice to help your loved one feel more comfortable with their therapy.

Monitoring and adjusting CPAP therapy for a loved one with dementia is a continuous process that involves regular check-ins, strategy adjustments, and professional support. By staying attentive to their needs and being flexible, you can ensure that the therapy remains practical and comfortable. This improves your loved one's health and well-being and enhances your caregiving experience.

External Oxygen

Understanding Pulmonary Disease

As an experienced hospice nurse, I'll do my best to explain these topics clearly and compassionately. Let's dive in:

Common Pulmonary Diseases in Older Adults

Pulmonary diseases affect the lungs and can make breathing difficult. As we age, our lungs become less efficient and more susceptible to these conditions.

Common pulmonary diseases in older adults include:

Disease	Description	Common Symptoms
Chronic Obstructive Pulmonary Disease (COPD)	A group of lung diseases that block airflow and make breathing difficult	Shortness of breath, chronic cough, wheezing
Pneumonia	An infection that inflames the air sacs in one or both lungs	Cough with phlegm, fever, chills, difficulty breathing
Pulmonary Fibrosis	Scarring of the lungs, which makes them stiff and rigid to expand	Shortness of breath, dry cough, fatigue
Lung Cancer	Uncontrolled growth of abnormal cells in one or both lungs	Persistent cough, coughing up blood, chest pain

These conditions can significantly impact quality of life and may require ongoing management, including oxygen therapy in some cases.

The Connection Between Dementia and Breathing Difficulties

When a loved one has both dementia and a pulmonary disease, it can create unique challenges. Here's why:

1. **Difficulty communicating symptoms:** People with dementia may struggle to express when they're having trouble breathing or experiencing discomfort.

2. **Increased confusion:** Low oxygen levels can worsen confusion and other cognitive symptoms in people with dementia.

3. **Challenges with treatment adherence:** Memory problems can make it hard for individuals to remember to use inhalers and oxygen or take medications as prescribed.

4. **Anxiety and agitation:** Breathing difficulties can cause anxiety, which may lead to agitation or behavioral changes in people with dementia.

5. **Increased risk of complications:** People with dementia may be less likely to notice or report early signs of respiratory infections, leading to more severe illness.

How you can help:

- Watch for non-verbal signs of breathing difficulties, such as rapid breathing, using accessory muscles, or blue-tinged lips or fingernails.

- Ensure a calm, well-ventilated environment.

- Help your loved one use prescribed treatments, such as inhalers or oxygen.

- Stay in close communication with their healthcare team.

Remember, caring for someone with both dementia and pulmonary disease can be challenging, but you're not alone. Don't hesitate to contact healthcare providers or support groups for help and guidance.

The Importance of Oxygen Therapy

I understand that caring for a loved one with dementia and pulmonary issues can be challenging. Let's discuss oxygen therapy, which can significantly improve your loved one's quality of life.

Why Oxygen is Prescribed

Oxygen is essential for every cell in our body to function correctly. When someone has a pulmonary disease, their lungs may not be able to get enough oxygen into the bloodstream, which is why doctors prescribe oxygen therapy.

Common reasons for oxygen prescription:

1. Low blood oxygen levels (hypoxemia)

2. Shortness of breath that impacts daily activities

3. Sleep-related breathing problems

4. To improve exercise tolerance

5. To reduce strain on the heart

It's crucial to understand that oxygen is a medication. It should only be used as a doctor prescribes, as too much oxygen can be harmful in some conditions.

Benefits of Oxygen Therapy for Dementia Patients

For individuals with both dementia and pulmonary disease, oxygen therapy can offer several significant benefits:

Benefit	Description	Impact on Dementia
Improved cognitive function	Better oxygenation of the brain	It may reduce confusion and improve alertness
Better sleep	It helps maintain oxygen levels during sleep	This can lead to improved mood and decreased agitation
Increased energy	More oxygen for the body's cells	It may increase the ability to participate in daily activities
Reduced strain on the heart	It requires less work for the heart to pump oxygenated blood	It can improve overall health and potentially slow disease progression
Decreased anxiety	Easier breathing can reduce feelings of panic	This may lead to calmer behavior and improved quality of life

It's important to note that while oxygen therapy can't cure dementia or pulmonary disease, it can significantly improve comfort and quality of life for your loved one.

Types of Oxygen Therapy (Nighttime, Post-Activity, Continuous)

Oxygen therapy can be prescribed in different ways, depending on your loved one's specific needs. Here are the main types:

1. **Nighttime Oxygen Therapy**

   o Used during sleep

   o Helps maintain oxygen levels when breathing naturally slows

   o May improve sleep quality and daytime alertness

2. **Post-Activity Oxygen Therapy**

- o Used after physical exertion

- o Helps recover oxygen levels after activities that cause shortness of breath

- o Can improve the ability to perform daily tasks

3. **Continuous Oxygen Therapy**

- o Used 24 hours a day

- o Necessary for those with consistently low oxygen levels

- o Provides constant support for breathing

Key points to remember about oxygen therapy:

- Always follow the doctor's prescription for when and how much oxygen to use

- Never change the oxygen flow rate without consulting the healthcare team

- Keep oxygen equipment clean and well-maintained

- Ensure backup power for electrical oxygen concentrators

- Follow safety precautions, as oxygen supports combustion

Caring for someone using oxygen therapy may seem overwhelming at first, but with time and practice, it will become a regular part of your routine. Remember, this therapy helps your loved one breathe easier and potentially improves their overall well-being.

If you have any concerns or questions about oxygen therapy, don't hesitate to contact your healthcare provider. They're there to support you and ensure the best care for your loved one.

Introduction to Nasal Cannulas

I understand that medical equipment can sometimes seem intimidating. Let's explore nasal cannulas, a typical and effective way to deliver oxygen therapy to your loved one with dementia and pulmonary issues.

What is a Nasal Cannula?

A nasal cannula is a simple, lightweight device that delivers oxygen to a person who needs breathing support. It consists of a few essential parts:

- **Tubing**: A long, flexible tube that connects to the oxygen source

- **Prongs**: Two short tubes that sit just inside the nostrils

- **Adjustable loop**: Goes behind the ears to keep the cannula in place

Key features of a nasal cannula:

- Typically made of soft, flexible plastic

- Available in different sizes to ensure comfort

- Can deliver oxygen at various flow rates, usually between 1-6 liters per minute

- Allows the wearer to eat, drink, and speak while receiving oxygen

How Nasal Cannulas Work

Nasal cannulas deliver a steady stream of oxygen-enriched air directly into the nostrils. Here's a step-by-step explanation of the process:

1. Oxygen flows from the source (tank or concentrator) through the tubing

2. The oxygen travels through the prongs into the nostrils

3. As the person breathes in, they inhale a mixture of room air and supplemental oxygen

4. This oxygen-rich air travels to the lungs, where it's absorbed into the bloodstream

5. The oxygenated blood then circulates throughout the body, supporting vital functions

It's important to note that nasal cannulas don't push oxygen into the lungs. Instead, they provide an oxygen-rich environment for normal breathing.

Advantages of Nasal Cannulas for Dementia Patients

Nasal cannulas offer several benefits that make them particularly suitable for individuals with dementia:

Advantage	Description	Why it's helpful for dementia patients
Comfort	Lightweight and less restrictive than masks	Less likely to cause agitation or confusion
Easy communication	It doesn't cover the mouth	Allows for clearer speech, which is vital for expressing needs
Simplicity	Easy to put on and take off	Reduces frustration for both patient and caregiver
Eating and drinking	Doesn't interfere with meals	Maintains everyday routines, which is comforting for dementia patients
Familiarity	It becomes part of the daily routine	It can provide a sense of security once the patient is used to it

Alternatives to Nasal Cannulas for Dementia Patients

While nasal cannulas are often the first choice, some alternatives might be more suitable in certain situations:

1. **Oxygen Masks**

   o Cover the nose and mouth

   o Can deliver higher oxygen concentrations

   o Useful for patients who need more oxygen than a cannula can provide

2. **Transtracheal Oxygen Therapy**

- o Oxygen is delivered directly into the windpipe through a small tube

- o Less visible, which some patients prefer

- o Requires a minor surgical procedure

3. **Oxygen Conserving Devices**

- o Deliver oxygen only when the patient inhales

- o Can extend the life of portable oxygen tanks

- o May be less effective for some patients with irregular breathing patterns

4. **Non-Invasive Ventilation (NIV)**

- o Uses a mask that covers the nose or nose and mouth

- o Provides pressurized air to help keep airways open

- o Often used for sleep apnea or severe COPD

Choosing the suitable oxygen delivery method:

- Consult with the healthcare team to determine the best option

- Consider your loved one's comfort and preferences

- Be prepared to try different methods to find the most effective one

- Remember that needs may change over time, requiring adjustments to the oxygen therapy plan

As a caregiver, your observations are invaluable. If you notice any issues with the nasal cannula or other oxygen delivery methods, such as skin irritation, frequent displacement, or signs that your loved one isn't getting enough oxygen (like increased confusion or shortness of breath), don't hesitate to contact the healthcare team.

Remember, the goal is to provide comfortable, effective oxygen therapy that improves your loved one's quality of life. With patience and proper care, oxygen therapy can become a routine part of daily life, helping your loved one breathe easier and potentially enhancing their overall well-being.

Encouraging Compliance with Oxygen Therapy

I've seen firsthand how challenging it can be to encourage loved ones with dementia to use their oxygen therapy consistently. Feeling frustrated or worried is normal when your family member resists something to help them. Let's explore why this happens and how you can help.

Understanding Resistance to Oxygen Use

Resistance to oxygen use is common, especially in individuals with dementia. Understanding the reasons behind this resistance can help you approach the situation with empathy and find practical solutions.

Common reasons for resistance:

- **Discomfort**: The nasal cannula might feel strange or irritating.

- **Confusion**: Your loved one may not understand why they need oxygen.

- **Fear**: The equipment might seem scary or overwhelming.

- **Loss of independence**: Oxygen therapy might make them feel more dependent or ill.

- **Forgetfulness**: They might forget to use it due to memory issues.

- **Embarrassment**: They may feel self-conscious about using oxygen in public.

Remember, your loved one isn't being difficult on purpose. Their behavior often results from their condition and how they're experiencing the world around them.

Strategies for Promoting Acceptance

Encouraging oxygen use requires patience, creativity, and a person-centered approach. Here are some strategies that can help:

1. **Educate gently**

   o   Explain the benefits of oxygen in simple terms

   o   Use visual aids if possible

   o   Repeat information as needed, staying patient and calm

2. **Make it routine**

   o   Incorporate oxygen use into daily activities

   o   Use reminders or cues in the environment

3. **Ensure comfort**

   o   Check that the cannula fits properly

   o   Use moisturizing gel or cream for nasal passages if needed

   o   Adjust room temperature and humidity for comfort

4. **Offer choices**

   o   Let them choose when to use oxygen (within doctor's recommendations)

   o   Allow them to pick the color of the cannula or tubing if possible

5. **Use distraction**

   o   Engage them in enjoyable activities while using oxygen

   o   Play their favorite music or TV shows during oxygen use

6. **Provide emotional support**

   o   Offer reassurance and encouragement

   o   Stay positive and celebrate small victories

7. **Consult healthcare providers**

   o   Discuss ongoing issues with the care team

   o   Consider adjustments to the oxygen therapy plan if needed

Creating a Positive Association with Oxygen Use

Creating positive associations can significantly improve compliance with oxygen therapy. Here are some ways to make oxygen use a more positive experience:

Strategy	Description	Example
Reward system	Offer small rewards for consistent use	A favorite snack or activity after using oxygen
Positive language	Use encouraging words and phrases	"The oxygen helps you feel stronger for our walk."
Comfort items	Pair oxygen use with comforting objects	A soft blanket or favorite chair during oxygen time
Social connection	Make oxygen time a chance for positive interaction	Reading together or looking at family photos
Sensory pleasures	Incorporate enjoyable sensory experiences	Aromatherapy or gentle hand massage during use

Additional tips for creating positive associations:

- **Be a role model**: Demonstrate a positive attitude towards the oxygen equipment.

- **Celebrate improvements**: Point out when they breathe easier or have more energy.

- **Make it familiar**: Decorate the oxygen equipment with favorite stickers or colors.

- **Use humor**: If appropriate for your loved one, gentle humor can lighten the mood.

Remember, every person is unique, and what works for one individual may not work for another. It's okay to try different approaches and adjust your strategies over time.

A note on safety and well-being:

While encouraging compliance is essential, balancing this with respect for your loved one's autonomy and dignity is crucial. If resistance to oxygen use is severe or causing significant distress, consult with the healthcare team. They can help assess whether the current oxygen therapy plan is the best option or if adjustments are needed.

As a caregiver, your role in supporting oxygen therapy is invaluable. Your patience, understanding, and creative problem-solving can make a real difference in your loved one's health and quality of life. Remember to also take care of yourself during this process. Caregiver support groups or counseling can be helpful resources as you navigate these challenges.

Respecting Dignity and Autonomy

I understand the delicate balance between providing necessary care and respecting your loved one's dignity and autonomy. This balance is vital when managing oxygen therapy. Let's explore how to maintain your loved one's sense of self while ensuring they receive the care they need.

The Importance of Dignity in Dementia Care

Dignity is a fundamental human right that doesn't diminish with age or cognitive decline. For individuals with dementia, maintaining dignity can significantly impact their quality of life and willingness to accept care.

Critical aspects of dignity in dementia care:

- **Respect**: Treating your loved one as an adult, not a child

- **Privacy**: Maintaining personal space and modesty

- **Identity**: Recognizing their individuality and life history

- **Comfort**: Ensuring physical and emotional well-being

- **Autonomy**: Allowing choices and control where possible

- **Communication**: Speaking to them, not about them, in their presence

Impact of preserving dignity:

1. Improved mood and behavior

2. Greater cooperation with care routines

3. Enhanced sense of self-worth

4. Better quality of life

5.   Stronger relationships with caregivers

Remember, even if your loved one can't express it, they can still feel and appreciate being treated with dignity.

Balancing Safety with Personal Choice

One of the biggest challenges in dementia care is balancing safety concerns with your loved one's desire for independence. This is especially true regarding oxygen therapy, which is crucial for health but can feel restrictive.

Strategies for finding balance:

Strategy	Description	Example
Assess risks	Evaluate potential dangers realistically	Is occasional non-use of oxygen genuinely harmful, or just not ideal?
Offer controlled choices	Provide options within safe parameters	"Would you like to use your oxygen in the living room or bedroom?"
Use assistive technology	Implement devices that promote safety and independence	Oxygen equipment with built-in safety features
Create a safe environment.	Modify the living space to allow more freedom	Secure oxygen tubing to prevent tripping hazards
Gradual adaptation	Introduce changes slowly to allow adjustment	Start with short periods of oxygen use and gradually increase

Remember: It's okay to allow your loved one to take small, calculated risks if it significantly improves their quality of life. Consult with healthcare providers to understand what risks are acceptable.

Involving Your Loved One in Decision-Making

Including your loved one in decisions about their care, including oxygen therapy, can help maintain their sense of control and improve cooperation. Here's how you can involve them:

1. **Simplify choices**

   o   Offer two or three clear options

   o   Use visual aids if helpful

   o   Allow extra time for decision-making

2. **Respect preferences**

   o   Listen to their concerns about oxygen use

   o   Try to accommodate preferences when it is safe to do so

   o   Acknowledge their feelings, even if you can't always act on them

3. **Encourage participation in care routines**

   o   Let them hold or touch equipment before use

   o   Guide them in putting on the nasal cannula if possible

   o   Involve them in cleaning or storing equipment

4. **Provide information**

   o   Explain procedures in simple terms

   o   Be honest about why oxygen is necessary

   o   Use analogies they can relate to (e.g., "Oxygen is like fuel for your body")

5. **Seek ongoing feedback**

   o   Regularly ask how they feel about their oxygen therapy

   o   Watch for non-verbal cues of discomfort or distress

   o   Be willing to revisit decisions and make changes

Tips for effective communication during decision-making:

- Use a calm, respectful tone

- Speak clearly and at a moderate pace

- Use simple language and short sentences

- Give one piece of information at a time

- Use a gentle touch to maintain focus, if appropriate

- Be patient and allow time for responses

A note on capacity:

It's essential to recognize that decision-making capacity can fluctuate in individuals with dementia. On good days, your loved one may be able to participate more fully in decisions. On other days, they may need more support. Always strive to include them to the extent possible, even if their input is limited.

Remember, involving your loved one in decisions about their care isn't just about the decisions themselves. It's about preserving their sense of self, respecting their personhood, and maintaining your relationship. Even minor involvements can make a big difference in how they perceive their care and their willingness to cooperate with necessary treatments like oxygen therapy.

By focusing on dignity, balancing safety with choice, and involving your loved one in decision-making, you're not just providing care – you're honoring their humanity. This approach can make the caregiving journey more rewarding for both of you, even amidst the challenges.

Setting Up the Oxygen Equipment

I understand that managing oxygen therapy can feel overwhelming. Let's break down some practical tips to make this aspect of caregiving more manageable and effective.

Proper setup of oxygen equipment is crucial for safety and effectiveness. Here's a step-by-step guide:

1. **Choose the right location**

   o Place the oxygen concentrator in a well-ventilated area

   o Keep it at least 6 feet away from heat sources or open flames

   o Ensure easy access for both the patient and caregiver

2. **Connect the equipment**

   o   Attach the tubing to the oxygen outlet

   o   Check that all connections are secure

   o   Ensure tubing is free of kinks or bends

3. **Set the flow rate**

   o   Adjust the liter flow as prescribed by the doctor

   o   Double-check the setting before each use

4. **Prepare the nasal cannula**

   o   Gently curve the prongs to fit comfortably in the nostrils

   o   Adjust the tubing to fit securely behind the ears

5. **Organize the space**

   o   Create a clear path for tubing to prevent tripping

   o   Use tubing holders or clips to keep lines tidy

   o   Have backup supplies readily available

Safety checklist:

☐ No smoking signs posted

☐ Fire extinguisher nearby

☐ Backup power source for electric concentrators

☐ Emergency contact numbers visible

☐ Spare nasal cannulas and tubing on hand

Ensuring Comfort During Oxygen Use

Comfort is critical to encouraging consistent oxygen use. Here are some tips to enhance comfort:

Area of Focus	Tips for Comfort
Nasal Care	- Apply water-based lubricant to nostrils - Use saline nasal spray to prevent dryness - Gently clean nostrils daily
Skin Care	- Pad tubing behind ears with soft material - Rotate pressure points regularly - Use skin barrier creams if needed
Humidity	- Consider using a humidifier in the room - Ensure adequate fluid intake - Use moisturizing lip balm
Temperature	- Keep room temperature moderate - Use lightweight, breathable bedding - Dress in comfortable, non-restrictive clothing

Additional comfort measures:

- Encourage regular position changes to prevent pressure sores

- Offer frequent sips of water to combat dry mouth

- Use pillows or cushions to support comfortable positioning

- Consider soft background music or nature sounds to create a relaxing atmosphere

Monitoring Oxygen Use and Effectiveness

Monitoring is essential to ensure your loved one receives the full benefit of oxygen therapy. Here's what to watch for:

1. **Physical signs of adequate oxygenation:**

   o Pink, warm skin tone

   o Normal breathing rate (12-20 breaths per minute for adults)

   o Ability to speak in complete sentences without breathlessness

   o Improved energy levels

2. **Signs that may indicate insufficient oxygen:**

   o   Bluish tint to lips, fingernails, or skin

   o   Rapid, shallow breathing

   o   Confusion or increased agitation

   o   Excessive drowsiness

3. **Equipment checks:**

   o   Confirm proper flow rate at each use

   o   Listen for unusual noises from the concentrator

   o   Check tubing and connections daily for wear or damage

   o   Clean or replace filters as recommended by the manufacturer

4. **Usage tracking:**

   o   Keep a log of daily oxygen use

   o   Note any issues or concerns

   o   Track changes in symptoms or behavior

Using a pulse oximeter:

If your healthcare provider recommends a pulse oximeter, it can be a helpful tool for monitoring oxygen levels at home.

- Normal oxygen saturation is typically 91% or higher; however, if your loved one has COPD, their normal oxygen saturation maybe 89% to 91%.

- Follow your doctor's guidelines for acceptable ranges; it is possible to poison someone with too much oxygen as well as cause respiratory arrest because your loved one's drive to breathe – due to the disease process – changed from lack of oxygen to a level of carbon dioxide.

- Record readings at different times of day and during various activities

When to seek medical help:

Contact your healthcare provider immediately if you notice:

- Persistent drop in oxygen saturation below prescribed levels

- Significant increase in shortness of breath

- Signs of respiratory infection (fever, increased cough, change in mucus color)

- Any sudden changes in mental status or level of consciousness

Remember, your observations are invaluable as a caregiver. Trust your instincts if something seems off, and don't hesitate to contact your healthcare team with concerns.

Caring for a loved one on oxygen therapy can be challenging, but with these practical tips, you can create a safer, more comfortable environment. Remember to also take care of yourself in the process. Regular breaks, support from family and friends, and open communication with your healthcare team can help you provide the best care possible for your loved one.

Managing Oxygen Therapy in Different Settings

I understand that managing oxygen therapy for your loved one with dementia can feel challenging, especially when moving between different settings. However, with proper planning and knowledge, you can ensure your family members receive the oxygen they need wherever they are. Let's explore how to manage oxygen therapy in various situations.

At Home

Home is where your loved one will likely spend most of their time, so it's crucial to create a safe and comfortable environment for oxygen use.

Critical considerations for home oxygen use:

1. **Safety first**

   o   Keep oxygen away from heat sources and open flames

o   Post "No Smoking" signs visibly

o   Ensure proper electrical setup for oxygen concentrators

2. **Organize the space**

o   Create a dedicated area for oxygen equipment

o   Use tubing organizers to prevent tripping hazards

o   Keep backup supplies in an easily accessible location

3. **Maintain equipment**

o   Clean or replace filters regularly

o   Check tubing and cannulas for wear and tear

o   Keep equipment dust-free

4. **Emergency preparedness**

o   Have a backup power source for electric concentrators

o   Keep emergency numbers visible

o   Create an evacuation plan that includes oxygen needs

Daily routine checklist:

☐   Check the oxygen flow rate

☐   Inspect tubing and connections

☐   Clean nasal cannula

☐   Monitor oxygen supply (for tank users)

☐   Record usage and any concerns

Remember, consistency is vital. Establishing a routine can help your loved one feel more comfortable with their oxygen therapy.

During Outings and Travel

Venturing outside the home with oxygen equipment might seem daunting, but with proper preparation, it can be manageable and even enjoyable.

Planning for outings:

Consideration	Actions to Take
Duration	Calculate oxygen needs based on time away.
Transportation	Secure oxygen tanks properly in vehicles.
Destination	Research oxygen-friendly locations.
Weather	Protect equipment from extreme temperatures.
Emergency	Bring contact info for oxygen suppliers at your destination.

Tips for successful outings:

- Use portable oxygen concentrators for greater mobility

- Bring extra batteries or charging equipment

- Pack a small bag with essential supplies (extra tubing, cannulas, etc.)

- Plan rest stops if traveling long distances

- Inform airlines, hotels, or event venues in advance about oxygen needs

Remember: Many people use oxygen in public. Encourage your loved one to feel confident about their needs and not let oxygen therapy limit their experiences.

In Healthcare Facilities

Transitions to healthcare facilities can be stressful, but proper communication can ensure continuity of care.

Preparing for facility visits or stays:

1. **Before arrival**

   - Inform the facility about oxygen needs

   - Provide current prescription and equipment details

   - Ask about their oxygen policies (Can you bring your own? Will they provide it?)

2. **During the stay**

   - Bring a copy of the oxygen prescription

   - Ensure staff are aware of your loved one's specific needs

   - Advocate for consistent oxygen use as prescribed

3. **For outpatient visits**

   - Bring portable oxygen if needed

   - Allow extra time for security checks if bringing oxygen equipment

   - Inform staff if oxygen levels typically drop during procedures

Communication is vital: Create a simple, straightforward document with your loved one's oxygen needs, including:

- Prescribed flow rate

- Type of equipment used

- Any specific instructions or preferences

- Your contact information

This can be invaluable for healthcare staff, especially if your loved one has difficulty communicating due to dementia.

Special considerations for dementia patients:

- Familiar items can provide comfort in new settings. Consider bringing a favorite blanket or photo.

- If possible, stay with your loved one to provide reassurance and assist with oxygen use.

- Inform staff about strategies to help your loved one accept oxygen therapy.

Managing oxygen therapy across different settings may seem complex, but with practice, it becomes easier. Remember, the goal is to ensure your loved one receives the oxygen they need while maintaining their quality of life. Feel free to ask for help or clarification from healthcare providers or oxygen suppliers. Your dedication to your loved one's care is admirable, and with the proper support and information, you can confidently manage their oxygen needs in any setting.

Addressing Common Concerns and Challenges

I understand that you may face various challenges. Let's explore some common concerns and practical solutions to help make this journey easier for you and your loved one.

Skin Irritation and Discomfort

Skin irritation is frequent for oxygen users, especially those with sensitive skin or who use oxygen for extended periods. Here's how to address this:

Common causes of skin irritation:

- Pressure from nasal cannula or tubing

- Dryness from oxygen flow

- Allergic reactions to equipment materials

- Moisture buildup under tubing

Solutions to prevent and treat skin irritation:

1. **Rotate contact points**

   o Adjust the position of the tubing slightly every few hours

   o Use both ears alternately to support tubing

2. **Protect the skin**

   o   Apply water-based moisturizer to contact areas

   o   Use soft padding or gauze behind ears and on cheeks

   o   Consider hypoallergenic tape to secure tubing

3. **Maintain cleanliness**

   o   Clean the nasal cannula daily with mild soap and water

   o   Pat the skin dry thoroughly after washing

4. **Address dryness**

   o   Use a humidifier with an oxygen system if approved by your provider

   o   Apply a water-based lubricant inside nostrils

Products that may help with skin irritation

Product Type	How It Helps	Example
Skin barrier cream	Creates a protective layer	Cavilon Barrier Cream
Nasal moisturizer	Reduces nasal dryness	Neilmed Nasogel
Cannula cushions	Softens contact points	Oxy-Soft Nasal Cushions
Ear protectors	Reduces pressure behind ears	Ear Buddies

If skin irritation persists or worsens, consult your healthcare provider. They may recommend alternative equipment or additional treatments.

Mobility Issues

Oxygen therapy doesn't have to mean being homebound. With the right approach, your loved one can maintain mobility and independence.

Strategies to improve mobility:

1. **Choose the right equipment**
   - Consider portable oxygen concentrators for outings
   - Use lightweight tanks for short trips
   - Explore backpack-style carriers for hands-free movement

2. **Organize the home environment**
   - Create clear pathways for tubing
   - Use wall-mounted tubing holders to keep lines off the floor
   - Consider a central oxygen system for larger homes

3. **Practice safe movement**
   - Teach your loved one to move with the oxygen, not against it
   - Use a walker or rollator with an attached oxygen holder
   - Ensure proper lighting to prevent tripping

4. **Plan for outings**
   - Calculate oxygen needs based on outing duration
   - Bring extra batteries or tanks
   - Know the locations of oxygen refill stations if traveling

Remember: Encouraging mobility, even if it's just moving around the house, can improve both physical and mental well-being for your loved one.

Social Stigma and Embarrassment

It's not uncommon for individuals using oxygen therapy to feel self-conscious, especially in public. Here's how you can help your loved one overcome these feelings:

Understanding the emotional impact:

- Fear of drawing attention

- Feeling different or "sick"

- Worry about being a burden

Ways to address social stigma and embarrassment:

1. **Educate and normalize**

   o Share facts about oxygen therapy with your loved one and others

   o Point out other people using oxygen in public or media

   o Remind them that oxygen is a tool for better health, like glasses or a cane

2. **Focus on benefits**

   o Highlight how oxygen therapy improves their quality of life

   o Encourage participation in activities they enjoy

   o Celebrate the independence that proper oxygen use allows

3. **Adapt social situations**

   o Plan shorter outings at first to build confidence

   o Choose oxygen-friendly venues and activities

   o Inform friends and family about oxygen needs to create a supportive environment

4. **Personalize the equipment**

   o Use colorful or patterned oxygen bags

   o Decorate the oxygen tank or concentrator (if safe to do so)

   o Choose fashionable or discreet carrying options

Empowering statements to use:

- "Oxygen helps you do the things you love."

- "Using oxygen shows you're taking control of your health."

- "Many people use oxygen – it's more common than you might think."

Remember: Your attitude towards oxygen use can significantly influence your loved one's perception. Approach it with positivity and normalcy.

Addressing these common concerns and challenges can significantly improve your loved one's experience with oxygen therapy. Always remember that you're not alone in this journey. Don't hesitate to contact healthcare providers, support groups, or other caregivers for additional advice and support. Your dedication to your loved one's care is commendable, and with patience and the right strategies, you can help them live a fulfilling life while managing their oxygen needs.

Safety Considerations

I understand that ensuring the safety of your loved one using oxygen therapy is a top priority. Safety considerations are crucial for your family member's well-being and your peace of mind. Let's explore some key safety aspects to remember when managing oxygen therapy at home.

Fire Safety with Oxygen Equipment

Oxygen supports combustion, making fire safety critical. Here are essential guidelines to follow:

Fire Safety Rules:

1. **No smoking:** Enforce a strict no-smoking policy in the home and around oxygen equipment.

2. **Keep away from heat sources:** Maintain a 5-foot distance between oxygen equipment and heat sources like radiators, space heaters, or fireplaces.

3. **Avoid flammable products:** Avoid petroleum-based products (e.g., Vaseline) near oxygen. Opt for water-based alternatives.

4. **Proper storage:** Store oxygen cylinders upright and secure them to prevent tipping.

5. **Electrical safety:** Use grounded outlets and avoid overloading circuits.

Important reminders:

- Post "No Smoking - Oxygen in Use" signs around the home

- Inform visitors about oxygen safety rules

- Keep a fire extinguisher easily accessible and know how to use it

Everyday Household Items to Keep Away from Oxygen

Item	Reason
Candles	Open flame
Hairspray	Flammable aerosol
Oil-based lotions	Flammable ingredients
Electric razors	Potential sparks
Synthetic fabrics	Can create static electricity

Remember, vigilance is critical in preventing fire hazards associated with oxygen use.

Preventing Falls and Accidents

Falls are a significant risk for individuals with dementia, and oxygen equipment can add to this risk. Here's how to minimize fall hazards:

Fall Prevention Strategies:

1. **Clear pathways:**

   o Remove clutter from floors

   o Secure loose rugs or remove them entirely

   o Organize oxygen tubing to prevent tripping

2. **Improve lighting:**

   - Ensure well-lit pathways, especially at night
   - Use nightlights in hallways and bathrooms

3. **Assistive devices:**

   - Consider a walker or rollator with an oxygen tank holder
   - Install grab bars in bathrooms and near stairs

4. **Proper footwear:**

   - Encourage wearing non-slip shoes or slippers
   - Avoid loose or backless footwear

5. **Equipment management:**

   - Use shorter oxygen tubing when possible
   - Consider a portable oxygen concentrator for increased mobility

Additional safety tips:

- Encourage regular exercise to maintain strength and balance (as approved by their doctor)
- Be extra cautious during transitions (e.g., getting up from a chair, entering/exiting the shower)
- Consider a medical alert system for quick assistance in case of a fall

Emergency Preparedness

Being prepared for emergencies is crucial when caring for someone on oxygen therapy. Here's how to stay ready:

Emergency Preparedness Checklist:

- ☐ Create an emergency contact list (including doctors, oxygen suppliers, and family members)

- ☐ Have a backup power source for electric oxygen concentrators

- ☐ Keep extra oxygen tanks on hand

- ☐ Prepare an emergency go-bag with essential supplies

- ☐ Develop and practice an evacuation plan that accounts for oxygen needs

What to include in your emergency go-bag:

- Copies of critical medical documents

- List of current medications

- Extra nasal cannulas and tubing

- Portable oxygen supply (if available)

- Basic first aid kit

- Flashlight and extra batteries

- Bottled water and non-perishable snacks

Types of Emergencies to Prepare For

Emergency Type	Specific Preparations
Power outage	Backup battery, generator, or extra oxygen tanks
Natural disaster	Evacuation plan, emergency supply kit
Medical emergency	List of medications, advance directives, emergency contacts
Equipment failure	Contact info for oxygen supplier, backup equipment

Important: Register with your local power company if your loved one requires electricity for their oxygen. Many utilities prioritize power restoration for homes with medical needs.

In case of emergency:

1. Stay calm

2. Ensure your loved one's safety first

3. Call for appropriate help (911, oxygen supplier, etc.)

4. Follow your prepared emergency plan

Being prepared can significantly reduce stress and ensure better outcomes in emergencies. Review and update your emergency plans and supplies regularly to stay ready.

Safety should always be your top priority when managing oxygen therapy at home. Following these fire safety, fall prevention, and emergency preparedness guidelines can create a safer environment for your loved one. Don't hesitate to contact healthcare providers or your oxygen supplier with any safety concerns or questions. Your dedication to your loved one's care is admirable, and with proper safety measures in place, you can provide them with the best possible care while using oxygen therapy.

Communicating with Healthcare Providers

I understand that effective communication with healthcare providers is crucial for ensuring the best care for your loved one with dementia who uses oxygen therapy. Your role as a caregiver is invaluable, and your observations and insights can greatly inform medical decisions. Let's explore how to communicate effectively with healthcare providers.

Important Information to Share

When speaking with healthcare providers, certain information is precious. Here's what you should be prepared to share:

Key Information Checklist:

- ☐ Changes in oxygen usage or effectiveness

- ☐ New or worsening symptoms

- ☐ Medication changes or side effects

- ☐ Eating and drinking habits

- ☐ Sleep patterns

- ☐ Mobility changes

- ☐ Cognitive changes or behaviors

- ☐ Any falls or accidents

Tip: Keep a daily log of these items. This can help you spot trends and provide accurate information to healthcare providers.

Information to Track Daily

Category	What to Note
Oxygen Use	Hours used, flow rate, any issues with equipment
Breathing	Shortness of breath, coughing, the color of lips/nails
Behavior	Confusion, agitation, sleep disturbances
Physical	Energy levels, appetite, mobility
Medications	Any missed doses, new side effects

Remember, no detail is too small. What might seem insignificant to you could be an essential clue for healthcare providers.

When to Seek Medical Attention

Knowing when to seek immediate medical attention can be crucial. Here are some situations that warrant prompt medical care:

Red Flags - Seek Immediate Medical Attention If:

1. **Breathing difficulties:**

    o   Severe shortness of breath, even with oxygen

    o   Bluish tint to lips, fingernails, or skin

2. **Changes in consciousness:**

    o   Unusual drowsiness or difficulty waking

    o   Sudden confusion or disorientation

3. **Physical symptoms:**

    o   Chest pain

    o   Rapid heart rate

    o   Fever above 101°F (38.3°C)

4. **Equipment issues:**

    o   Oxygen equipment malfunction that can't be quickly resolved

5. **Falls:**

    o   Any fall, especially if there's a head injury or prolonged time on the floor

Important: Trust your instincts. If you're worried, seeking medical attention and being reassured is better than waiting and risking complications.

Advocating for Your Loved One's Needs

As a caregiver, you are your loved one's voice. Advocating for their needs is an integral part of your role. Here's how to do it effectively:

Tips for Effective Advocacy:

1. **Be prepared:**
   - o Bring your logs and notes to appointments
   - o Write down questions in advance
   - o Bring a list of current medications

2. **Communicate clearly:**
   - o Be specific about your concerns
   - o Use concrete examples
   - o Don't downplay symptoms or challenges

3. **Ask questions:**
   - o If you don't understand something, ask for clarification
   - o Request explanations in layman's terms if medical jargon is confusing

4. **Follow up:**
   - o Take notes during appointments
   - o Ask about next steps and follow-up plans
   - o Request written instructions when possible

5. **Seek second opinions when necessary:**
   - o If you're unsure about a diagnosis or treatment plan, it's okay to seek another professional opinion

Assertive Communication Techniques:

- Use "I" statements, such as "I've noticed..." or "I'm concerned about..."

- Be specific: Instead of "Mom isn't doing well," say, "Mom has been more short of breath this week and has used her oxygen for two extra hours each day."

- Ask for clarification: "Can you explain why you recommend this change?"

- Express your needs: "I need more information about managing these new symptoms."

Remember: You are essential to your loved one's care team. Your insights and concerns are valuable and should be taken seriously by healthcare providers.

Effective communication with healthcare providers can significantly improve the care your loved one receives. You play a crucial role in managing their health and well-being by sharing important information, recognizing when to seek immediate care, and advocating for their needs.

Feel free to speak up or ask questions. Healthcare providers appreciate engaged caregivers actively involved in their loved ones' care. Your dedication and attention to detail can make a real difference in the quality of care your family member receives.

Remember to take care of yourself too. Caregiving can be challenging, and asking for support or resources for yourself is okay. Your well-being is essential; taking care of yourself allows you to provide the best care for your loved one.

Preparing for End-of-Life Decisions

While difficult to contemplate, preparing for end-of-life decisions is essential to caregiving. Having these conversations and making plans can provide peace of mind and ensure your loved one's wishes are respected.

Steps in Preparing for End-of-Life Decisions:

1. **Start the Conversation**

   o Choose a calm moment to discuss end-of-life wishes with your loved one.

   o Approach the topic with sensitivity and openness.

2. **Understand Your Loved One's Wishes**

   o Discuss preferences for medical interventions, pain management, and place of care.

   o Explore spiritual or cultural considerations.

3. **Document Decisions**

   o Ensure advance directives (living will, healthcare power of attorney) are in place.

   o Consider creating a POLST (Physician Orders for Life-Sustaining Treatment) form.

4. **Communicate with Healthcare Providers**

   o Share documented wishes with all relevant healthcare providers.

   o Ensure copies of advance directives are in medical records.

5. **Plan for Practical Matters**

   o Discuss funeral or memorial preferences.

   o Address financial and legal matters (wills, estate planning).

6. **Prepare Emotionally**

  - o Seek support from counselors, support groups, or spiritual advisors.

  - o Allow yourself to process emotions as you plan.

7. **Focus on Quality of Life**

  - o Discuss what quality of life means to your loved one.

  - o Align care decisions with these values.

End-of-Life Consideration	Questions to Discuss	Documentation Needed
Medical Interventions	Preferences for resuscitation, ventilation, feeding tubes	Living Will, POLST Form
Pain Management	Comfort goals, medication preferences	Advance Directive, Pain Management Plan
Place of Care	Preference for home, hospital, or hospice care	Documented in Advance Care Plan
Spiritual/Cultural Needs	Desired rituals, religious support	Noted in Personal Directive

Remember, coping with grief and loss is a profoundly personal journey. There's no right or wrong way to feel; seeking help is okay. By acknowledging your grief, finding meaning in your caregiving role, and preparing for difficult decisions, you're honoring both yourself and your loved one.

These conversations and preparations, while challenging, can bring a sense of peace and allow you to focus on creating meaningful moments with your loved one. Don't hesitate to lean on your support network, seek professional help if needed, and be gentle with yourself throughout this process. Your role as a caregiver is invaluable, and taking care of your emotional well-being is essential to providing compassionate care.

When to Consider Hospice

Hospice care is a compassionate approach to end-of-life care that focuses on comfort, quality of life, and dignity. It's important to understand that choosing hospice doesn't mean giving up – it means shifting the focus from curative treatment to comfort care.

Critical aspects of hospice care include:

1. Pain management and symptom control

2. Emotional and spiritual support for the patient and family

3. Assistance with personal care and daily living activities

4. Respite care for family caregivers

5. Bereavement support for loved ones

Hospice care is typically provided by a team of professionals, including:

- Doctors

- Nurses

- Social workers

- Chaplains or spiritual advisors

- Trained volunteers

Hospice Service	Description
Medical Care	Pain management, symptom control, and medication management.
Personal Care	Assistance with bathing, dressing, and other daily activities.
Emotional Support	Counseling for patient and family, addressing fears and concerns.
Spiritual Care	Support for spiritual needs and end-of-life rituals.
Practical Support	Help with household tasks, errands, and respite care.

The importance of timely hospice involvement

Deciding when to involve hospice care can be emotionally challenging, but **early involvement often leads to better outcomes** for both the person with dementia and their caregivers. Here's why timely hospice care is crucial:

1. **Improved quality of life**: Hospice teams are experts in managing pain and other symptoms, helping your loved one feel more comfortable.

2. **Reduced hospitalizations**: Proper symptom management often reduces the need for emergency room visits or hospital stays.

3. **Emotional and spiritual support**: Hospice offers counseling and support services that benefit you and your loved one.

4. **Time to say goodbye**: Earlier involvement gives family members more time to spend with their loved one and address unfinished business.

5. **Caregiver support**: Hospice provides education, resources, and respite care to help you navigate this challenging time.

Remember, choosing hospice doesn't mean death is imminent. Many patients receive hospice care for months, allowing them to make the most of their remaining time with improved comfort and quality of life.

Benefits of Early Hospice Involvement	Impact on Patient and Family
Better symptom management	Increased comfort and reduced suffering
Comprehensive support	Improved overall quality of life for the patient and caregivers
Avoid crises	Less stress and anxiety for family members
Time for meaningful moments	Opportunity to create lasting memories and say goodbyes

By understanding dementia, hospice care, and the benefits of timely involvement, you're better equipped to make informed decisions about your loved one's care. Remember, you're not alone in this journey – hospice teams are there to support both you and your loved one every step of the way.

Signs It May Be Time for Hospice Care

As a caregiver or family member of someone with dementia, recognizing when it's time to consider hospice care can be challenging. This decision is deeply personal and often emotional. However, certain signs can help guide you in making this vital choice. Let's explore these indicators in detail.

Physical indicators

Physical changes are often the most noticeable signs that your loved one's condition is progressing. **Look for these physical indicators**:

1. **Significant weight loss**: A 10% or more decrease in body weight in six months.

2. **Frequent infections**: Pneumonia or urinary tract infections that are becoming harder to treat.

3. **Difficulty swallowing**: This can lead to choking, coughing during meals, or refusal to eat.

4. **Increased pain**: Despite efforts to manage it with medication.

5. **Skin breakdown**: Pressure sores or other skin issues that aren't healing.

6. **Changes in breathing**: Shortness of breath, labored breathing, or long pauses between breaths.

7. **Decreased mobility**: Becoming bed-bound or unable to sit up without support.

Physical Indicator	What to Look For
Weight Loss	Loose clothing, visible bone structure, sunken cheeks
Swallowing Difficulties	Coughing during meals, holding food in the mouth, refusing to eat
Skin Issues	Redness, open sores, slow healing of wounds
Mobility Changes	Inability to walk independently, frequent falls, reluctance to move

Cognitive and behavioral changes

As dementia progresses, you may notice significant changes in your loved one's cognitive abilities and behavior. **Fundamental changes to watch for include**:

- Increased confusion and disorientation

- Difficulty recognizing family members

- Loss of ability to communicate verbally

- Agitation, aggression, or combative behavior

- Withdrawal from social interactions

- Changes in sleep patterns (sleeping more during the day, restless at night)

- Hallucinations or delusions

Remember, these changes can be distressing for you and your loved one. Hospice care can help you manage these symptoms and improve your quality of life.

Frequent hospitalizations or ER visits

If you find yourself taking your loved one to the emergency room or hospital more often, it might be time to consider hospice care. **Signs to consider include**:

1. Multiple hospitalizations within the past six months

2. Recurring infections or illnesses

3. Increasing difficulty managing symptoms at home

4. Longer recovery times after each hospital stay

Frequency of Medical Visits	Consideration
1-2 ER visits in 6 months	Monitor closely and consult with a doctor.
3+ ER visits in 6 months	This is a strong indication for a hospice evaluation.
Any hospital stay longer than one week	Consider hospice discussion.

Decline in daily functioning

A significant decline in your loved one's ability to perform daily tasks independently is a strong indicator that hospice care may be beneficial. **Watch for**:

- Inability to dress, bathe, or groom without assistance

- Incontinence or loss of bladder and bowel control

- Difficulty moving from bed to chair without help

- Inability to prepare or eat meals independently

- Decreased interest in previously enjoyed activities

These changes often mean that your loved one requires more intensive care, which hospice can provide while ensuring comfort and dignity.

In conclusion, deciding when to consider hospice care is complex and personal. By being aware of these signs – physical changes, cognitive decline, frequent hospitalizations, and decreased daily functioning – you can make a more informed choice about when to seek additional support. Remember, hospice care is not about giving up hope; it's about ensuring the best possible quality of life for your loved one and support for you as a caregiver.

The Benefits of Hospice Care for Dementia Patients

When considering hospice care for your loved one with dementia, it's essential to understand the numerous benefits this specialized care can provide. Hospice focuses on comfort and quality of life, offering a holistic approach to supporting the patient and their family. Let's explore these benefits in detail.

Pain management and symptom control

One of the primary goals of hospice care is to ensure that your loved one is as comfortable as possible. **Effective pain management and symptom control can significantly improve their quality of life.**

Critical aspects of pain and symptom management in hospice care include:

1. **Personalized pain assessment**: Hospice professionals are trained to recognize pain in patients who cannot communicate verbally.

2. **Tailored medication plans**: Medications are carefully selected and adjusted to provide maximum comfort with minimal side effects.

3. **Non-pharmacological interventions** may include massage, music therapy, or aromatherapy to complement medication.

4. **Regular monitoring**: The hospice team assesses the patient's comfort level and adjusts care as needed.

5. **Management of other symptoms**: This includes addressing issues like shortness of breath, nausea, anxiety, and sleep disturbances.

Common Dementia Symptoms	Hospice Management Approach
Pain	Tailored pain medication, positioning, gentle massage
Agitation	Calming techniques, environmental adjustments, medication if necessary
Difficulty swallowing	Dietary modifications, proper positioning, oral care
Skin issues	Regular repositioning, specialized mattresses, wound care

Emotional and spiritual support

Hospice care recognizes that emotional and spiritual well-being is as important as physical comfort. **This holistic approach can provide immense comfort to the patient and their family.**

Emotional and spiritual support in hospice care includes:

- Counseling services for the patient and family members

- Support from social workers to address practical and emotional concerns

- Chaplain services for spiritual support, regardless of religious affiliation

- Assistance with life review and legacy projects

- Grief counseling for family members, both before and after their loved one's passing

Remember, this support is tailored to your family's needs and beliefs. The hospice team is there to provide comfort and guidance, not to impose any particular spiritual or religious views.

Respite care for family caregivers

Caring for a loved one with dementia can be physically and emotionally exhausting. **Hospice care recognizes the vital role of family caregivers and offers respite services to prevent burnout.**

Respite care benefits include:

1. Short-term relief from caregiving duties

2. Opportunity for self-care and rest

3. Time to attend to personal matters or other family responsibilities

4. Professional care for your loved one, ensuring their needs are met

5. Reduced stress and improved overall well-being for the caregiver

Improved quality of life

The ultimate goal of hospice care is to improve the patient's and their family's overall quality of life. **This is achieved through expert care, support, and a focus on comfort rather than curative treatments.**

Ways hospice care can improve quality of life:

- Allowing the patient to remain in familiar surroundings, often at home

- Providing equipment and supplies necessary for comfort and care

- Offering 24/7 support and guidance for family caregivers

- Facilitating meaningful interactions and moments between the patient and their loved ones

- Ensuring dignity and respect in all aspects of care

Addressing not just physical needs but also emotional, social, and spiritual needs Quality of Life Aspect	Hospice Care Impact
Comfort	Reduced pain and distressing symptoms.
Dignity	Personalized care respecting individual preferences.
Family connection	Support for meaningful interactions and memory-making.
Peace of mind	24/7 professional support and guidance.

In conclusion, hospice care offers numerous benefits for dementia patients and their families. By focusing on comprehensive symptom management, providing emotional and spiritual support, offering respite care, and striving to improve overall quality of life, hospice care can make a significant difference in your loved one's final months or years.

Remember, choosing hospice care doesn't mean giving up hope. Instead, it means shifting the focus to ensuring the best possible quality of life and comfort for your loved one. It's about making the most of your time together, creating meaningful moments, and finding peace in knowing your loved one receives expert, compassionate care.

Common Misconceptions About Hospice Care

When considering hospice care for a loved one with dementia, you may encounter several misconceptions that can cause hesitation or concern. Understanding the realities of hospice care is essential to making an informed decision. Let's address the most common misconceptions and clarify what hospice care entails.

Hospice is not giving up.

One of the most pervasive misconceptions about hospice care is that it means "giving up" on your loved one. **This couldn't be further from the truth.**

Here's why hospice is not giving up:

1. **Shift in focus**: Hospice represents a change in care goals, not an abandonment of care. The focus shifts from curative treatments to comfort and quality of life.

2. **Active care**: Hospice provides expert care to manage symptoms and improve comfort.

3. **A holistic approach** addresses not just physical needs but also emotional, social, and spiritual aspects of well-being.

4. **Empowerment**: Hospice empowers patients and families to make choices about their care and how they want to spend their remaining time.

5. **Celebration of life**: Many hospice programs encourage life reviews and legacy projects, which celebrate the person's life and accomplishments.

Misconception	Reality
Hospice means no more treatment.	Hospice provides active treatment for symptoms and comfort.
Choosing hospice means giving up hope.	Hospice shifts hope to quality of life and meaningful moments.
Hospice is only for the last few days of life.	Hospice can provide care for months, enhancing life quality.

Hospice doesn't mean imminent death.

Another common misconception is that hospice care is only for the last few days or weeks of life. **Hospice care can be beneficial for months and sometimes even longer.**

Key points to understand:

- Hospice eligibility typically requires a prognosis of six months or less, but this is not a strict limit.

- Many patients receive hospice care for several months, with some even "graduating" from hospice if their condition stabilizes.

- Earlier involvement of hospice often leads to a better quality of life and can sometimes even extend life by reducing stress on the body.

- Hospice care can be discontinued if the patient's condition improves or if they decide to pursue curative treatments again.

Time in Hospice	Potential Benefits
Days to weeks	Immediate comfort care and family support in crisis
Weeks to months	Sustained symptom management, quality time with family
Months or longer	Long-term comfort, potential for stabilization or improvement

Hospice care can be provided at home.

Many people believe that choosing hospice care means their loved one must move to a facility. **Hospice care is often provided right in the comfort of the patient's home.**

Understanding home hospice care:

1. **Flexibility**: Hospice care can be provided wherever the patient calls home – private residences, assisted living facilities, or nursing homes.

2. **Customized care**: The hospice team works with you to create a care plan that fits your home environment and family dynamics.

3. **Equipment and supplies**: Necessary medical equipment (like hospital beds or oxygen) is provided and set up in the home.

4. **24/7 support**: While the hospice team isn't present 24/7, they're always available by phone for guidance and can visit as needed.

5. **Family involvement**: Home hospice allows family members to be intimately involved in care, with guidance from the hospice team.

6. **Familiar surroundings**: Patients often find comfort surrounded by familiar sights, sounds, and loved ones.

Aspect of Care	In-Home Hospice Provision
Medical care	Regular visits from nurses and doctors
Personal care	Assistance with bathing and dressing by hospice aides
Emotional support	Visits from social workers and counselors
Spiritual care	Chaplain visits if desired

It's important to note that while home hospice is common, inpatient hospice facilities are available for those who need or prefer that option. Some patients may transition between home and inpatient care as their needs change.

In conclusion, understanding these common misconceptions about hospice care can help you make a more informed decision for your loved one with dementia. Hospice is not about giving up or waiting for death; it's about living life as fully and comfortably as possible in whatever time remains. It offers expert care that can often be provided at home, surrounding your loved one with familiar comforts and loving family members.

Remember, choosing hospice care is a profoundly personal decision. It's okay to have questions and concerns. Don't hesitate to contact hospice providers in your area to learn more about their services and how they might benefit your loved one and your family. Your choice to consider hospice care demonstrates your commitment to ensuring the best possible quality of life for your loved one, which is an act of profound love and care.

How to Initiate the Hospice Conversation

Initiating a conversation about hospice care can be challenging and emotionally charged. However, having these discussions early can lead to better care decisions and more time to prepare. Here's how to approach this sensitive topic with compassion and clarity.

Talking with your loved one

When possible, it's essential to involve your loved one with dementia in the decision-making process. While their ability to participate may vary, including them shows respect for their wishes and autonomy.

Tips for talking with your loved one:

1. **Choose the right time and place**: Find a quiet, comfortable setting where your loved one is most alert and receptive.

2. **Be direct but gentle**: Use clear, simple language. Avoid euphemisms that might confuse them.

3. **Listen actively**: Pay attention to their verbal and non-verbal responses.

4. **Respect their feelings**: Acknowledge any fears or concerns they express.

5. **Focus on the benefits**: Explain how hospice can help manage their symptoms and improve comfort.

6. **Be patient.** This may need to be an ongoing conversation. Don't rush to decide everything in one sitting.

Use visual aids: If appropriate, consider using brochures or videos to help explain hospice care. What to Say	What to Avoid
"I want to talk about how we can keep you comfortable."	"We need to discuss end-of-life care."
"Hospice can help us manage your pain better."	"There's nothing more we can do for you."
"What's most important to you right now?"	"You should consider hospice care."

Discussing with family members

Bringing up hospice care with other family members can sometimes be as challenging as discussing it with your loved one. Family dynamics, differing opinions, and emotional responses can complicate these conversations.

Strategies for family discussions:

- **Plan**: Consider who should be part of the conversation and how to involve distant family members.

- **Choose a spokesperson**: Designate one person to lead the conversation if helpful.

- **Share information**: Before the discussion, provide educational materials about hospice care to all family members.

- **Be inclusive**: Ensure everyone has a chance to express their thoughts and feelings.

- **Focus on your loved one's wishes**: If known, center the discussion on what your loved one with dementia would want.

- **Address concerns**: Be open to questions and address fears or misconceptions about hospice care.

Seek professional help: Consider involving a social worker or counselor to facilitate the conversation if family conflicts arise. **Common Family Concerns**	Possible Responses
"Isn't this giving up?"	"Hospice focuses on quality of life and comfort, not giving up."
"It's too soon to consider hospice."	"Earlier hospice involvement often leads to better care and support."
"We can't afford it."	"Medicare, Medicaid, and most private insurances usually cover hospice."

Consulting with healthcare providers

Healthcare providers play a crucial role in the decision to pursue hospice care. They can provide valuable insights into your loved one's condition and prognosis and help you understand if hospice is appropriate.

Steps for consulting healthcare providers:

1. **Schedule a dedicated appointment**: Request a meeting to discuss your loved one's care options, including hospice.

2. **Prepare questions**: Write down your questions and concerns beforehand. Some key questions might include:

   - Is my loved one eligible for hospice care?

   - How might hospice benefit them at this stage?

   - What changes in their condition should we be watching for?

3. **Bring support**: Consider having another family member present to help remember information.

4. **Take notes**: Write down important points or ask if you can record the conversation for future reference.

5. **Discuss prognosis**: While difficult, understanding the expected progression of your loved one's condition can help you make decisions.

6. **Ask about referrals**: If hospice seems appropriate, ask for referrals to reputable hospice providers in your area.

7. **Follow-up**: Don't hesitate to contact the healthcare provider with any additional questions after the meeting.

Healthcare Provider	Role in Hospice Discussion
Primary Care Physician	Overall health assessment and long-term care planning.
Neurologist	Dementia progression and symptom management.
Geriatrician	Specialized care needs for older adults.
Palliative Care Specialist	Expert in comfort care and quality of life issues.

Remember, initiating the hospice conversation is an act of love and care. It shows that you're thinking proactively about ensuring the best possible quality of life for your loved one. While these discussions can be difficult, they often bring a sense of relief and clarity once they're underway.

It's normal to feel a range of emotions during this process. Don't hesitate to seek support for yourself, whether from friends, support groups, or professional counselors. Taking care of your emotional well-being is crucial as you navigate this challenging journey.

Ultimately, the goal is to make informed decisions that honor your loved one's wishes and provide them with the most appropriate and compassionate care possible. By approaching these conversations with openness, empathy, and a focus on your loved one's well-being, you can navigate this critical decision-making process with greater confidence and peace of mind.

The Hospice Evaluation Process

Understanding the hospice evaluation process can help alleviate some of the anxiety and uncertainty you may feel when considering this option for your loved one with dementia. This process ensures that hospice care is appropriate and tailored to your loved one's specific needs. Let's explore each step in detail.

Eligibility criteria for dementia patients

Specific criteria apply to people with dementia who are eligible for hospice care. **These criteria are guidelines, and each case is evaluated individually**.

Key eligibility factors for dementia patients include:

1. **Disease progression**: The person should be in the late stages of dementia, typically stage 7, on the Functional Assessment Staging Test (FAST).

2. **Functional decline**: Inability to perform daily activities without substantial assistance.

3. **Medical complications**: Presence of conditions such as aspiration pneumonia, upper urinary tract infections, sepsis, or multiple stage 3-4 pressure ulcers.

4. **Nutritional decline**: Difficulty eating and swallowing, leading to weight loss.

5. **Verbal communication**: Limited to fewer than six intelligible daily words.

6. **Mobility**: Unable to walk without assistance and eventually becoming bed-bound.

Eligibility Factor	Description
FAST Stage 7	Very severe cognitive decline, minimal verbal communication
ADL Dependence	Requires help with most or all activities of daily living
Medical Complications	Recurrent infections, difficulty swallowing, pressure sores
Nutritional Decline	Significant weight loss, difficulty eating independently

Remember, meeting these criteria doesn't automatically mean hospice is the right choice, nor does failing to meet all requirements necessarily disqualify someone. The decision involves a comprehensive evaluation by healthcare professionals and discussions with the family.

What to expect during the evaluation

The hospice evaluation is a thorough process designed to assess your loved one's needs and determine whether hospice care is appropriate. **It is typically provided at no cost and does not obligate you to choose hospice care**.

The evaluation process usually includes:

- **Initial consultation**: A hospice representative will meet with you and your loved one to explain services and answer questions.

- **Medical review**: The hospice team will review your loved one's medical history and condition.

- **Physical assessment**: A nurse will conduct a physical examination to evaluate symptoms and care needs.

- **Psychosocial assessment**: A social worker may assess emotional needs and family dynamics.

- **Home safety evaluation**: If care will be provided at home, the team will assess the environment for safety and equipment needs.

- **Discussion of goals**: The team will discuss your loved one's care goals and preferences with you.

Evaluation Step	Conducted By
Initial Consultation	Hospice Representative
Medical Review	Hospice Physician
Physical Assessment	Hospice Nurse
Psychosocial Assessment	Social Worker

Creating a care plan

If your loved one is found eligible for hospice and you decide to proceed, the next step is creating a personalized care plan. This plan is a **collaborative effort** between the hospice team, your loved one (if able to participate), and your family.

The care plan typically includes:

1. **Symptom management strategies**: Plans for managing pain, anxiety, breathing difficulties, and other symptoms.

2. **Medication regimen**: A review and adjustment of current medications, focusing on comfort and symptom control.

3. **Personal care routines**: Plans for bathing, feeding, and other daily care needs.

4. **Emotional and spiritual support**: Arrange counseling, chaplain visits, or other support services.

5. **Family education**: Training for family caregivers on providing care and recognizing important signs or symptoms.

6. **Emergency procedures**: Clear instructions on what to do in case of emergencies or sudden changes in condition.

7. **Respite care arrangements**: Plans for providing breaks to family caregivers.

Care Plan Component	Purpose
Symptom Management	Ensure comfort and quality of life.
Medication Management	Optimize effectiveness and minimize side effects.
Personal Care	Maintain dignity and prevent complications.
Emotional Support	Address the psychological needs of the patient and family.

It's important to understand that the care plan is a **dynamic document**. It will be regularly reviewed and adjusted as your loved one's needs change. You and your family will be integral parts of this ongoing process.

Remember, the hospice evaluation and care planning process ensures your loved one receives the most appropriate and compassionate care possible. It's an opportunity to ask questions, express concerns, and actively participate in shaping your loved one's care.

Don't hesitate to ask for clarification if anything is unclear during this process. The hospice team supports you and your loved one every step of the way. They aim to honor your loved one's wishes, provide expert care, and help your entire family through this challenging time.

By understanding and actively participating in the evaluation and care planning process, you're taking an essential step in ensuring the best possible care and quality of life for your loved one with dementia. While sometimes emotional, this process can also bring relief and clarity as you navigate this difficult journey.

Preparing for Hospice Care

Once you've decided to pursue hospice care for your loved one with dementia, there are several important steps to take to ensure a smooth transition. This preparation phase is crucial for creating a supportive environment and understanding what to expect. Let's explore these steps in detail.

Choosing a Hospice Provider

Selecting the right hospice provider is a critical decision that can significantly impact the quality of care your loved one receives. **Take your time with this process, and don't hesitate to ask questions.**

Consider the following when choosing a hospice provider:

1. **Certification and accreditation**: Ensure the provider is Medicare-certified and, ideally, accredited by a national organization.

2. **Range of services**: Look for providers offering comprehensive medical, emotional, and spiritual support.

3. **Availability**: Choose a provider that offers 24/7 emergency on-call services.

4. **Experience with dementia**: Ask about their specific experience in caring for patients with dementia.

5. **Staff qualifications**: Inquire about the training and qualifications of their care team members.

6. **Respite care options**: Check if they offer respite care to give family caregivers breaks.

7. **Bereavement support**: Look for providers that offer grief counseling and support after your loved one's passing.

Question to Ask	Why It's Important
How quickly can you start services?	Ensures timely care initiation
What is your staff-to-patient ratio?	Indicates the level of individual attention
How do you manage pain in dementia patients?	Reveals expertise in dementia-specific care
What support do you offer family caregivers?	Indicates the level of family involvement and support

Setting up the care environment

Creating a safe, comfortable environment is essential for hospice care, especially if your loved one will be cared for at home. **The goal is to promote comfort, safety, and ease of care.**

Critical considerations for setting up the care environment:

- **Bedroom setup**: Ensure the bed is accessible from both sides. If recommended by the hospice team, consider a hospital bed.

- **Bathroom modifications**: Install grab bars, a raised toilet seat, and non-slip mats if needed.

- **Clear pathways**: Remove clutter and ensure clear paths for easy movement, primarily if a wheelchair or walker is used.

- **Lighting**: Provide adequate lighting to prevent falls and aid in care tasks.

- **Comfortable seating**: Have a comfortable chair for your loved one and seating for visitors.

- **Temperature control**: Ensure the room can be kept at a comfortable temperature.

- **Meaningful objects**: Include photos, favorite blankets, or other cherished items to create a comforting atmosphere.

Item	Purpose
Hospital bed	Allows for positioning adjustments, easier care
Bedside commode	Reduces the need for bathroom trips
Over-bed table	Provides surface for meals, activities
Night light	Improves safety during nighttime care

Understanding your role as a caregiver

As a family caregiver, your role will evolve with the introduction of hospice care. **While the hospice team will provide expert care, your involvement remains crucial.**

Your role as a caregiver may include:

1. **Being an advocate**: You know your loved one best. Share insights about their preferences, behaviors, and needs with the hospice team.

2. **Providing comfort**: Your presence and touch can be incredibly comforting. Spend time with your loved one, hold their hand, or sit with them.

3. **Assisting with personal care**: The hospice team will guide you in helping with feeding, bathing, or repositioning.

4. **Medication management**: While the hospice team will manage medications, you may be involved in administering them.

5. **Emotional support**: Provide reassurance and emotional support to your loved one.

6. **Communication liaison**: Keep other family members informed about your loved one's condition and care.

7. **Self-care**: Remember to take care of yourself too. Accept help
    and take breaks when needed.

Caregiver Task	Hospice Team Support
Personal care assistance	Training on safe techniques, along with regular help from hospice aides
Medication administration	Clear instructions, regular check-ins, 24/7 phone support
Emotional support	Counseling services, tips for communication
Recognizing changes in condition	Education on what to watch for, when to call for help

Remember, the hospice team supports you and your loved one. **Don't hesitate to ask for help or clarification when you need it.** They can provide training, answer questions, and support you as you navigate this new role.

Preparing for hospice care can feel overwhelming, but taking these steps can help create a smoother transition. By choosing the right provider, setting up a comfortable environment, and understanding your role, you're laying the groundwork for compassionate, quality care for your loved one.

This preparation phase is also a time for emotional readiness. It's normal to feel a mix of emotions – relief, sadness, anxiety, or even guilt. Remember that choosing hospice care is an act of love, focusing on comfort and quality of life for your loved one. Don't hesitate to lean on the hospice team, friends, or support groups for emotional support.

By taking these steps to prepare, you're ensuring that your loved one will receive the best possible care in their final stage of life while also setting yourself up to be an informed and supported caregiver. Your dedication to this process is a testament to your love and commitment to your family member's well-being.

Navigating the Emotional Journey

The decision to pursue hospice care for a loved one with dementia marks the beginning of a profound emotional journey. This period can be filled with complex feelings and challenges. Understanding these emotions and finding coping methods is crucial for you and your loved one. Let's explore this journey and discuss strategies for navigating it with resilience and grace.

Coping with grief and anticipatory loss

Grief is a natural response to loss, and it often begins well before the actual passing of a loved one. This is known as anticipatory grief. **Recognizing and acknowledging these feelings is an essential step in coping with them.**

Common experiences of anticipatory grief include:

- Sadness and tearfulness

- Anxiety about the future

- Anger or frustration

- Guilt over past events or current feelings

- A sense of helplessness

- Difficulty concentrating

- Physical symptoms like fatigue or changes in appetite

Strategies for coping with anticipatory grief:

1. **Acknowledge your feelings**: Allow yourself to feel whatever emotions arise without judgment.

2. **Share your feelings**: Talk to trusted friends, family members, or a professional counselor.

3. **Practice self-compassion**: Be kind to yourself. Grief is a normal and valid response to your situation.

4. **Stay connected**: Maintain relationships with friends and family. Don't isolate yourself.

5. **Take care of your physical health**: Eat well, exercise, and get enough sleep.

6. **Find healthy outlets**: Engage in activities that help you process your emotions, such as journaling, art, or music.

7. **Stay present**: While worrying about the future is natural, focus on the present moment and your time with your loved one.

Grief Response	Coping Strategy
Overwhelming sadness	Allow yourself to cry; talk to a supportive friend.
Anxiety about the future	Practice mindfulness; focus on one day at a time.
Guilt over negative feelings	Practice self-compassion; join a support group.
Physical exhaustion	Prioritize self-care; ask for help with tasks.

Finding support for caregivers

Caring for a loved one with dementia in hospice care can be emotionally and physically demanding. **Seeking support is not a sign of weakness but a necessary step in maintaining your well-being.**

Options for caregiver support include:

- **Support groups**: Join groups specifically for dementia caregivers or hospice families. These can be in-person or online.

- **Professional counseling**: Consider individual therapy to process emotions and develop coping strategies.

- **Respite care**: Take your hospice provider's respite services for necessary breaks.

- **Family and friends**: Don't hesitate to ask for and accept help from your support network.

- **Educational resources**: Attend workshops or webinars about caregiving and end-of-life care to feel more prepared.

- **Spiritual or religious support**: If applicable, seek guidance from spiritual leaders or faith communities.

- **Self-care activities**: Engage in activities that recharge you, even for short periods.

Type of Support	Benefits
Caregiver support groups	Shared experiences, practical tips, emotional validation.
Professional counseling	Personalized coping strategies and safe space to process emotions.
Respite care	Time for self-care and reduced burnout risk.
Educational resources	Increased confidence in caregiving, better preparedness.

Celebrating life and creating meaningful moments

While this time is undoubtedly challenging, it also presents opportunities to celebrate your loved one's life and create lasting memories. **Focusing on positive experiences can provide comfort and meaning during this challenging journey.**

Ideas for creating meaningful moments:

1. **Life review**: Remember happy memories, perhaps creating a scrapbook or memory box together.

2. **Music therapy**: Play your loved one's favorite songs or hymns. Music can often evoke positive responses, even in late-stage dementia.

3. **Sensory experiences**: Engage the senses with familiar scents, textures, or flavors that bring comfort.

4. **Nature connection**: If possible, spend time outdoors or bring nature inside with flowers or plants.

5. **Gentle touch**: Hold hands, give a soft massage, or sit close to provide comfort through touch.

6. **Family gatherings**: Organize small, quiet gatherings of close family and friends to share stories and love.

7. **Legacy projects**: Create something together that can be shared with future generations, like a recipe book or family tree.

8. **Spiritual practices**: If prayer, meditation, or other spiritual practices are essential to your loved one, engage in them.

Meaningful Activity	Potential Benefits
Looking at old photos	Stimulates memories and encourages storytelling.
Listening to favorite music	It evokes emotions and may improve mood.
Gentle hand massage	It provides comfort and promotes relaxation.
Reading aloud familiar stories	Offers comfort and maintains connection.

Remember, the goal is not to create grand gestures but to find moments of connection, comfort, and joy, however small they seem.

Navigating the emotional journey of hospice care for a loved one with dementia is undoubtedly challenging. It's a path filled with complex emotions, difficult decisions, and profound moments of love and connection. You can find strength and moments of peace by acknowledging your feelings, seeking support, and focusing on creating meaningful experiences.

It's important to remember that there's no "right" way to feel or grieve. Your journey is unique, and having good and bad days is okay. Be patient and compassionate with yourself as you navigate this path.

Lastly, don't forget that the hospice team supports you and your loved one. They can provide resources, counseling, and guidance to help you through this emotional journey. You're not alone in this process; reaching out for help when needed is a sign of strength and love for yourself and your loved one.

Legal and Financial Considerations

When caring for a loved one with dementia who is entering hospice care, it's important to consider legal and financial matters. These can be challenging topics, but planning can bring peace of mind and help avoid problems later. Let's look at some key things to consider.

Advance Directives and Power of Attorney

Advance directives say what kind of medical care your loved one wants if they can't speak for themselves. There are two main types:

1. Living Will: This document states what medical treatments your loved one wants or doesn't want at the end of life.

2. Healthcare Power of Attorney: This names someone to make medical decisions if your loved one can't.

Power of attorney is also crucial for money matters. It lets someone manage your loved one's finances if they can't do it themselves.

Why these papers matter:

- They make sure your loved one's wishes are followed

- They can prevent family arguments about care decisions

- They make it easier to handle bills and other money matters

Setting these up early is best while your loved one can still make decisions. If you haven't done this yet, talk to a lawyer who knows about elder law as soon as possible.

Document	What It Does
Living Will	States end-of-life care wishes
Healthcare Power of Attorney	Names someone to make medical decisions
Financial Power of Attorney	Names someone to handle money matters

Understanding Hospice Coverage and Costs

The good news is that Medicare, Medicaid, and most private insurance plans usually cover hospice care. This coverage includes:

- Doctor and nursing services

- Medical equipment and supplies

- Medications for symptom control and pain relief

- Short-term inpatient care, if needed

- Grief counseling for the patient and family

What's not covered:

- Room and board if the patient is at home or in a nursing facility

- Treatments aimed at curing the illness (instead of comfort care); such treatments can invalidate hospice services.

It's good to check with your hospice provider and insurance company to understand what's covered and what you might need to pay for.

Usually Covered	Usually Not Covered
Hospice team visits	Curative treatments (which can invalidate hospice services)
Medical equipment	Room and board at home
Medications for comfort	Care from providers outside the hospice

Additional Resources and Support Programs

Besides insurance, other programs might help with costs or provide extra support:

1. Veterans Benefits: If your loved one served in the military, they might qualify for special hospice benefits through the VA.

2. Social Security: Your loved one might be eligible for disability benefits if they're under 65.

3. Local Senior Services: Many communities have programs that offer seniors meals, transportation, or other help.

4. Alzheimer's Association: They offer support groups and education and can help you find local resources.

5. Area Agency on Aging: This government program can connect you with services in your area.

Don't be afraid to ask for help. Social workers at the hospice or your local senior center can often recommend programs that might help.

Resource	What It Offers
Veterans Benefits	Special hospice care for veterans
Social Security	Possible disability benefits
Alzheimer's Association	Support groups and education

Remember, dealing with legal and money matters can feel overwhelming, but it's integral to caring for your loved one. Don't hesitate to ask for help from professionals like lawyers, financial advisors, or social workers. They can guide you through these complex issues and help you make the best decisions for your family.

Conclusion

As we conclude ***CPAP and Oxygen for Dementia: A Dementia Care Essentials Guide***, it is essential to reflect on the profound journey of caregiving for a loved one with dementia. This path is filled with challenges and marked by moments of deep connection and love. Throughout this guide, we've explored practical strategies and compassionate approaches to managing CPAP and oxygen therapy to enhance patients' and caregivers' quality of life.

Remember, the heart of caregiving lies in empathy and understanding. While the road may be demanding, your dedication and resilience make a significant difference in your loved one's life. Embrace the support of healthcare professionals, community resources, and fellow caregivers as you navigate this journey. You are not alone; together, we can create a compassionate environment that honors dignity and autonomy.

As you move forward, continue to prioritize self-care and seek moments of joy and reflection. Celebrate the small victories and cherish the meaningful connections you build. Your role is invaluable, and your efforts are a testament to your love and commitment to your loved one.

Thank you for your unwavering dedication and kindness. May this guide serve as a source of support and empowerment, helping you provide the best possible care with compassion and grace.

Resources

Associations

Alzheimer's Association at https://www.alz.org/

Dementia Society of America at http://www.dementiasociety.org

National Institute on Aging at https://www.nia.nih.gov/

National Alliance for Caregiving at http://www.caregiving.org

Family Caregiver Alliance at http://www.caregiver.org

American Sleep Apnea Association at https://www.sleepapnea.org/

Author Bio

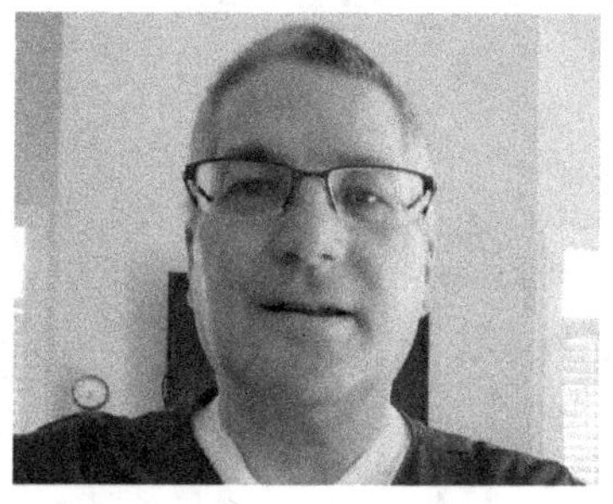

Peter Abraham, BSN, RN is an experienced nurse dedicated to supporting nurses, caregivers, families, and patients in their learning, growth, and well-being journey. Peter's nursing path encompasses practical experience as a cardiac telemetry nurse in a bustling cardiology unit at a Magnet-awarded teaching hospital. Additionally, Peter has fulfilled the role of a second-shift RN supervisor, overseeing an entire building in an SNF/LTC (Skilled Nursing Facility/Long-Term Care) setting with 151 residents. Remarkably, during the initial wave of COVID-19, the facility achieved an impressive close-to-100% recovery rate before operation warp speed was complete.

Furthermore, Peter's nursing career extends to rural home hospice care. As a visiting hospice registered nurse case manager, he offers compassionate care to patients in various settings, including private homes, personal care homes, assisted living facilities, skilled nursing facilities, and hospitals.

Moreover, Peter's desire to help others extends beyond his physical presence. At CompassionCrossing.Info, he writes articles to empower caregivers, family members, and fellow nurses in end-of-life care. Peter's drive to help others, which flows from his love of Christ Jesus, is a source of support and encouragement for all he reaches.

Other books by Peter Abraham include the following:

Empowering Excellence in Hospice: A Nurse's Toolkit for Best Practices series:

> Compliance-based, Eligibility Driven Hospice Documentation: Tips for Hospice Nurses
> Whispers of Time: Understanding the End-of-Life Timeline
> Terminal Clarity: Hospice Eligibility Guide for Nurses

Compassionate Caregiving series:

> Daily Hospice Care Planner: Organize, Communicate, and Provide Consistent Care
> Dignity in Dying: A Thoughtful Approach to Voluntary Stopping Eating and Drinking
> Palliative Sedation: A Compassionate Approach
> Hospice Medication Handbook: A Caregiver's Guide to Comfort Medications

Dementia Caregivers Essentials series:

> CPAP and Oxygen for Dementia
> Diabetes Care for Dementia
> Hallucination Management for Dementia
> Medication Compliance for Dementia
> Nutrition for Dementia
> Placement for Dementia
> Sundowning Management for Dementia

Connect with Peter On:

Website: https://compassioncrossing.info/